WORKOUT ROUTINES FOR MEN

Complete step-by-step guide for beginners to get in shape for the rest of your life with simple workouts and healty eating.

By

MASSIMO PRETE

Copyright ©2020 by Massimo Prete.
All rights reserved.

No part of this guide may be reproduced in any form without permission in writing from the publisher except in the case of brief quotations embodied in critical articles or reviews.

Legal & Disclaimer

The publisher and the author are providing this book and its contents on an "as is" basis and make no representations or warranties of any kind with respect to this book or its contents. The publisher and the author disclaim all such representations and warranties, including but not limited to warranties of healthcare for a particular purpose. In addition, the publisher and the author assume no responsibility for errors, inaccuracies, omissions, or any other inconsistencies herein.

The content of this book is for informational purposes only and is not intended to diagnose, treat, cure, or prevent any condition or disease. You understand that this book is not intended as a substitute for consultation with a licensed practitioner. Please consult with your own physician or healthcare specialist regarding the suggestions and recommendations made in this book. The use of this book implies your acceptance of this disclaimer.

The publisher and the author make no guarantees concerning the level of success you may experience by following the advice and strategies contained in this book, and you accept the risk that results will differ for each individual. The testimonials and examples provided in this book show exceptional results, which may not apply to the average reader, and are not intended to represent or guarantee that you will achieve the same or similar results.

The publisher and the author strongly recommend that you consult with your physician before beginning any exercise program. You should be in good physical condition and be able to participate in the exercise. The author is not a licensed healthcare care provider and represents that they have no expertise in diagnosing, examining, or treating medical conditions of any kind, or in determining the effect of any specific exercise on a medical condition.

You should understand that when participating in any exercise or exercise program, there is the possibility of physical injury. If you engage in this exercise or exercise program, you agree that you do so at your own risk, are voluntarily participating in these activities, assume all risk of injury to yourself, and agree to release and discharge the publisher and the author from any and all claims or causes of action, known or unknown, arising out of the contents of this book.

The publisher and the author advise you to take full responsibility for your safety and know your limits. Before practicing the skills described in this book, be sure that your equipment is well maintained and do not take risks beyond your level of experience, aptitude, training, and comfort level.

TABLE OF CONTENT

INTRODUCTION

I am very happy that you have chosen this book. If you like it, leave me a review on amazon, your opinion matters a lot to me.

The number 1 objective of this guide is, above all, to clarify your ideas on the concept of fitness, which is often equivalent to the ideal muscle definition.

In particular having a firm belly and sculpted abs.

I have the presumption to think that, at least in part, you don't have a clear idea of what you need to do to have good-looking abs.

That can't be your fault. In these times of information "saturation", of people who, in order to speculate, are ready to tell you a lot of lies, the web is full (and not only...).

I don't.

I will tell you the truth, in fact everything you will learn in this guide is not something I "invented", but the result of studies (of others, I have done their studies) and direct experiences: see my abdominal definition demonstrations on my site.

From all this, comes my method to achieve the goal of tortoise abs and a fit physique.

The information I'm about to give you is very important, simply because it's the only one that will really lead you to the result, in the shortest possible time and in full health, without hunger diets, hours of training and pills or various junk food.

You will have a clear idea of what you have to do immediately and especially how to do it, in fact, I will accompany you on your path and explain step by step working particularly on your head, your biggest obstacle.

In a few months (or even a few weeks) looking at your sculpted body you will feel satisfied with your efforts, you will have more confidence in yourself and will improve your relationship with others, appearing more attractive in the eyes of your partner.

To achieve this precious goal, turn off every distraction around you, throw yourself into reading and let's see in detail what you have to do.

WORKOUT SYSTEM TO GET IN SHAPE FOR EVER.

Let's start with the abs.

You know those unfair advertisements where they present abdominal equipment, describing them as miraculous solutions to superfluous fat?

They're freaking me out. In fact, it doesn't work that way!

Um... maybe you're wondering why I'm talking about fat, belly and slimming. In a few lines, it will become much clearer.

It's not necessarily that you are aware of having fat (maybe you don't really have any, I'll help you to understand it soon...) that prevents your abs from "showing up"...

"Indeed Max! I'm already thin, I only have a little bit of fat on my belly."

If you are certain that you need to reduce your weight, you should fix the following sentence firmly in your mind:

<u>If you have fat, even a little, on your abdomen, you'll be able to do 1000 abs a day, and they'll never come out!!!!</u>

Abdominals are muscles like any other, with the right training, they tone up, but working only abdominal exercises will never eliminate fat on your belly.

From this, we can easily understand that it is useless to do hundreds of sit-ups as the only solution to have them.

If you only train like this and do nothing else, you will never see your abs.

On the other hand, if you're sure you don't have a single strand of fat on your belly, there can only be two reasons...:

1. You have untrained abs, so they're unnoticeable.

2. You belong to that % of people who genetically have ligaments that hold together the abdominal muscles a little 'soft (lassi) and therefore, although they are trained and toned, do not form the classic squares.

In the first case, you can solve the problem by following a series of exercises to tone your body and in particular the super effective abdominals of this book, without having to worry about adjusting your diet and following a specific aerobic (and mixed aerobic/anaerobic) work to increase your metabolism.

In the second case, I am sorry to tell you that you will not be able to see a square abdomen. But don't beat yourself up, thanks to the above mentioned routine, you will be able to highlight the central groove as much as possible and develop your lateral muscles in the best possible way, definitely improving the general aesthetics of your abdomen.

That's good. I was particularly interested in this clarification. Now, let's see the 3 points from which nothing is left out that we are going to analyze in this book.

I'll be honest, if I had to do a percentage in order of importance, to have a good abdominal shape you need:

- 40% a strategic aerobic training that accelerates the metabolism.

- 50% a balanced, healthy and extremely clean diet.

- 10% a good routine for the tone of the whole body.

- But this 100% turns into 0% if your mind

is not ready.

Without too many words, you'll have to be 100% mentally strong to be able to face training and nutrition, i.e. 100% of the program.

I add that, if you do 50% of what I recommend, you will have to expect 50% of the results, in fact, you will most likely get little or nothing.

To summarize and simplify (in fact I was a bit twisted) you will have to be there 100% with your head and you will have to follow 100% of my advice. Only then will you be on the right track.

The meaning of being 100% in your head, if you had to reduce everything to just 4 steps, would be:

1. Trust my advice.

2. Trust yourself, convince yourself that nothing is impossible.

3. Focus on your goal, whether you're training or eating or going out for an evening at a restaurant or an aperitif.

4. Always plan your week, whether it's food or training: take a moment on Sunday

evening or Monday and, depending on your schedule, set up your training day by day.

Hold on a second.

The very first thing to do is the one I pointed out to you in step four.

To make this task easier for you, I have created a special chapter in which I have collected the material that I have always used and given to my clients. You can take advantage of the tables that I have prepared for you (you can find them at the bottom of the book, in the "Operating Materials" section).

Well, the foreword I made to you was a must. Also because I am absolutely convinced that to change one's life story and habits, it is necessary to understand why things happen.

But now, let's get down to business. In the next chapter, I'll start explaining what you have to start from and later on, what are the training routines to tone the whole body to make it defined and muscular.

SIMPLE WARM UPS

When starting a new workout routine, it can be easy to neglect proper warm up practices. We tend to get caught up in the actual exercise and jump right into them without a second thought. You may not notice it at first, but forgoing proper warm ups can cause serious damage to your muscles and joints in the long term. But don't let this fact scare you. Let it motivate you to warm up before *any* physical activity.

How many times have you jumped into a workout all pumped up and ready to go, only to feel a sharp pain, pull, or strain somewhere in your body? These pains are a direct result of not properly warming up. You always need to prepare your body before throwing it into motion.

Some people feel as though it's a waste of time to warm up, or unnecessary to do so *every single time* they want to work out. But these preventable aches and pains can lead to injuries or even long term conditions down the line.

A proper warm up will gently loosen up the body for whatever activity you are about to perform.

These movements will gradually increase your heart rate and help circulate blood to your muscles. This will loosen your joints and increase blood flow to the areas you are about to use.

Types of Warm Ups

Your warm up should include various movements, each one targeting a certain function in your body. These include cardiovascular exercises, stretch exercises, and strength exercises. The cardiovascular exercises will gradually increase your heart rate, causing your temperature to rise. As your blood temperature rises, oxygen becomes more readily available to working muscles, which may improve your endurance levels. You will feel your heart pumping, and that's a good sign; it's preparing for the work ahead.

The stretch exercises will loosen up your joints and wake up your muscles. Working out in the morning or after a long day at work means your muscles and joints will still be a little stiff. Stretch exercises will ensure that you don't pull or strain any muscles during your workout. Stretching properly warms the muscles and allows your large joints (specifically your shoulders and knees) the chance to move within their maximum ranges. During your warm up, your muscles will stretch and shrink, reducing the chance of tearing or pulling later.

The strength exercises (which should be done when the muscles are already warm) will help you slowly increase the level of intensity within your body's movements. These are usually done in bursts and will be highlighted below. During these warm ups, your breathing will get faster, your muscles will work harder, and your joints will get ready for more weight being placed on them.

These three types of exercises will help ease your body into the state you are about to put it into. The goal is never to shock your body into high energy activities. You always want to give your body a chance to loosen up and prepare itself for the work ahead. Your heart, lungs, and muscles will thank you for it.

Remember, warming up isn't just for your body. Taking the time to prepare for exercise also strengthens your mental focus and determination. Warming up gives your mind time to clear itself of distractions and think of the task ahead. Your mind needs to transition into exercise mode just as much as your body. Use this time to foster positive thinking and energy that will propel you forward. Many people even use warm up time as a chance to go over strategies, skills, techniques, and goals they want to reach during their workout. Always ensure that the transition into exercise is a holistic one; for the body and mind.

A Simple Warm Up Routine

Warming up doesn't need to be intimidating or complicated- in fact, warm ups can be both easy to do *and* entirely beneficial. Here are some simple warm ups that you can easily implement into any exercise regimen...

Each of the following moves should be done for 30 seconds, with no rest between moves. At the end of the routine, rest for 60 seconds then repeat from the top. Feel free to add these warm ups to an existing routine, perform them in any order, or to alter them completely. Anything goes, as long as you're moving!

1. The Jumping Jack

Many of us associate the jumping jacks with grade school gym class; however, they are the perfect way to start a simple warm up. In case you need reminding here are the directions on how to perform the ideal jumping jack:

Stand with your back straight and feet together. Make sure your core is engaged, and your hands are flat at your sides.

Jump and open your legs sideways, so the distance between your two feet is wider than your hips. Do the same with your arms and clap your hands above your head.

Jump back into the starting position.

Perform these motions repeatedly. Start off slow at first, then increase the speed.

This exercise is a great way to start pumping blood throughout the body. Your pulse and breathing will quicken, kicking things into motion.

2. Toe Taps

There are several ways to touch your toes, but

some are more beneficial than others. Instead of standing in one spot and reaching down to touch your toes, you should try something different.

First, stand with your feet apart and your arms at your sides.

Swing your left leg up to hip height (no higher) and, at the same time, bring your right arm to tap your left toes.

Return to starting position and repeat, this time with the opposite leg.

Swing your right leg up and touch the toes with your left leg.

Alternate between the two sides in a smooth, continuous way.

This particular toe touch may be difficult for those first starting out as it requires a certain degree of flexibility. However, this warm up does wonders even when done so incompletely. It may be difficult at first, but practice makes perfect.

This warm up will stretch the muscles along the back of both of your legs. These are the primary muscles you use when you run and should be warmed up before any physical activity.

Additionally, this warm up will loosen up the flexibility of your back, arms, and legs. The alternating pattern will ensure that all your limbs are ready to go.

3. Hip Circles

These hip circles will give you a time to catch your breath in between the more energy-intensive warm ups.

First, stand with your feet together. It usually helps to place your hands on your hips.

Raise your left knee to a 90-degree angle. Circle the hip out and make a huge circle with your knee. Make sure this movement is as wide as possible- without losing balance.

Repeat this 8 times before switching the direction.

Now, do the same but rotate the new inwards.

Once you've finished those 8, switch to your right left and repeat.

This particular exercise is done to loosen up the hips. Your hips support the weight of your body and are responsible for all movement in your upper leg. It is vital that you loosen up these joints for the upcoming workout.

4. Arm circles

Arm circles are similar to the hip circles, just for your upper body. These will loosen up any tension in your shoulders as well as gently stretch your muscles.

Begin with your feet shoulder-width apart and your arms on your sides.

Slowly make a full circle with your two arms, going forwards, down, back, and up.

Continue this circular motion for 8 repetitions.

Once complete, do the same in the opposite direction for another 8 rotations.

Soon you will feel your shoulders loosening up. You may even feel some joints crack- that is a good thing.

5. Jump Rope

Getting out your jump rope is one of the easiest ways to get your body energized before a workout. For best results, jump rope for two minutes at a consistent pace.

This warm up is easy: simply grab your jump rope and jump for two minutes.

Not only will jumping rope get your heart rate up, it will warm up your arms and shoulders, too!

Additionally, jumping rope doesn't need to be stationary and boring. You can change up this warm up however you see fit! If you have the space, you can run while jumping; you can go backward, you can even get fancy with the way you swing the rope. Nothing is off limits.

6. Walk Outs

This warm up is great for stretching out your hamstrings and activating your core.

Begin with your feet apart and your hands at your sides.

Bend at your hips and reach for the floor.

Slowly crawl out into a high plank position.

Once in this position, pause for a few seconds, then crawl backward.

When your hands are at your feet, stand up.

Repeat this 8 times.

Walk outs will work on your flexibility (reaching down to touch the floor), mobility (bending and crawling), as well as strength (holding up your body with your arms). If you feel ready, you can even pick up the pace to get your heart rate up.

Tips for Warming Up

Despite the simplicity of warming up, there are still some tips that are good to keep in mind- especially if you are a beginner.

First, keep it short. Remember that there is such a thing as over stretching. You should be warming up within the range of 15 to 30 minutes (depending on the intensity of your exercise to come). Any less won't help you with your workout, and any more will tire you out. Keep it simple, and keep it short. If you find that one particular warm up tires you out, remove it from your regimen. The more often you warm up, the better you will know what works best for you.

Similarly, tailor your warm ups. The warm up you do before a jog should be different from the one you do before lifting weights. The goal of your warm ups is to gradually increase the intensity from resting levels to moving levels.

Exercises such as yoga or pilates should be prepared for with neck rolls and pelvis twists. Alternatively, weight lifting should be prepared for with more intensive motion exercises. Take note of what muscles and body parts are needed for each activity, so you can warm up accordingly. Not only will this aid your body, but it will also keep things interesting.

Next, avoid static warm ups. Your warm ups should encourage continuous motions, however small, so that you're never standing still. Don't sit on the floor, lean over one leg, and stretch. This can actually increase the risk of injury. Instead, do stretches that involve dynamic movements. You may be stretching your leg, for example, but your whole body should be in motion. Make sure; somehow, your whole body is being incorporated into the warm up. The 6 warm ups listed above are great examples of this.

Lastly, focus. Use your warm up time to focus and motivate yourself. Exercising isn't easy for everyone, so take the time to hype yourself up. This can be as simple as closing your eyes and taking a few deep breaths. Or, it can be as complex as setting specific goals you want to reach. Warming up doesn't need to be daunting, difficult, or boring. It can be simple, easy, and even enjoyable.

ACCELERATE YOUR METABOLISM WITH FITNESSMAX METHOD TRAINING.

The very first thing you need to do is a self-assessment and figure out the amount of fat on your belly.

There is absolutely no point in having a well-trained and toned abdomen if you have a tummy! Believe me, it takes very little (even just a roll) to mist up your abs. This will indicate that even the rest of your body is not perfectly defined.

90% of the time, the solution is to lose that little bit of fat: this explains the sudden transformation that I documented in the demonstrations of 2009 and 2013. In fact, by reducing your fat mass to a minimum, your muscles will be more "visible", precisely because there will be nothing (or almost nothing) between the muscle and the skin.

That's why, I'll show you below, a good program to lose weight.

The best method, in my opinion, is to follow a

program of aerobic training and workouts to tone the whole body.

This simple strategy will gradually increase your metabolism, which, translated, means that your body will consume more energy throughout the day (yes, even while you sleep).

As a result, following a clean diet will lead to optimal weight loss.

Often, after an initial weight loss (mainly due to reduced water retention) this last process is not so immediate, especially if your bad habits are rooted in time.

If we put in a good dose of misinformation, many people give up, perhaps a step away from "unlocking", with the conviction that it is impossible for them.

But with the right dietary strategies and effective training planning, the results are guaranteed!

Your current level of training will influence the length of your journey and what grade you'll have to start from.

In this regard, if you've never trained or had any consistency in the last month, I've prepared a simple preparation sheet for you that will allow you, as soon as you're ready, to tackle short but intense workouts (IT, HIIT and the like) which, combined with a total body muscle tone workout, will allow you to increase your metabolism by significantly reducing your waistline.

If at the same time, you have trained your abs with the right strategy, you will be pleasantly surprised at the final result and will be able to show off a well-defined abdomen.

But as I told you at the beginning of this paragraph, as a first step, you will have to estimate how much fat is present on your belly.

Step 1: How much belly do I have? Fat Test.

This step is very important because it will allow you to understand how long you can expect to see your abdominals sculpted and consequently a defined body musculature.

Of course, it will take you as many weeks as you've got a few extra pounds.

To give you a sure reference, I go back a few years, to my 2013 demonstration of slimming and muscle definition. I was 32 years old at the time and I lost almost 8 kg in about 2 months. That was the time needed to reach a top level of fitness and definition.

Some of the people I have followed over time as a Personal Trainer Online have done even better, losing up to 10 kg in 2 months, but overall the average was about 1 kg per week.

But back to us. And in doing so, I'll tell you right now that weight isn't the only parameter you'll have to keep under control, in fact, it's not even the best!

The body circumferences in cm will be your allies to better control your progress.

In particular, the waist is a good parameter to keep an eye on if you want to get the turtle out of its shell.

Always from the analysis of the data I have available, the average waist drop is around 10 cm per 8 kg of weight lost in 2 months.

Just the waist is one of the most important parameters of the "test" that I will help you to do to find out approximately how many kg you have in excess.

Without shoes and clothes:

- Evaluate your weight and height.

- Measure your waist: with measuring tape, measure the narrowest point of your waist, usually a few inches above your navel. Help yourself by proceeding in front of a mirror.

- Measure your neckline just below Adam's apple.

- Enter this data in a spreadsheet (e.g. excel) applying this formula:

- FM Men (%) : 495 / {1.0324 - 0.19077 [log(neck waist)] + 0.15456 [log(stature)]-450

- You will have obtained a result in percentage.

The minimum % to hope for a well sculpted abdominal is about 9-10 %.

Suppose you weigh 80 kg and the result of your fat mass was 17 %. To get to 10 %, you'll have 7 % fat mass to remove, then:

80 x 7% = about 5.6 kg to lose.

In this case, we can assume 6 weeks of the program before you see your abdominals well sculpted.

Step 2: Structure your training program.

Here we go. Test in hand, you now need to know the next step in relation to the result:

The test result is equal to or less than 10 %.

You don't have a lot of fat and with well-trained muscles, you should get a great result..

Solution

Just follow the "Workout Routines Next Level" tab of this book. Please read the note that emphasizes the **"NO FAT"** version.

In your case, aerobic work is only recommended for general wellbeing and for maintaining fat mass at its current level.

If you want to reduce your fat mass by %, then follow the complete cycle in this report.

Estimated time

3-6 weeks for a tangible and concrete result.

Concrete yes, but note well that you should have a muscular body combined with abs, at least athletic (physical type "swimmer").

Most likely, if you bought this report but have such low fat, you will also have very little muscle mass.

In this condition, the risk is that you will appear toned in the abdomen, but with an excessively thin, not exactly attractive, "rickets" figure.

In this case, I advise you to take a path of increasing muscle mass, which requires a little more time and strategies different from those of this book.

To learn more, you can take advantage of the guides on my FitnessMax.it website, starting from the article/guide **"Training to increase mass: the best strategies"** (Italian Content.)

The test gave you a result of 11 to 15%.

You've got about 1 to 3 kg to lose.

Solution

Follow the Workout Routines Next Level.

Estimated time

3 to 6 weeks for a concrete result.

BUT HOW MAX? SAME TIME AS THOSE WHO ARE ALREADY SLIM?

Yeah.

In fact, following the complete program, you will lose fat and at the same time, you will tone your abdomen to the maximum, so the timing is still the same!

The test gave you a result of 15 to 20%.

In this case, you've got about 4 to 8 kg of fat to lose.

Solution

Especially if you haven't been training for months, extend the preparatory program that I will show you in the " Workout Routines for beginner" section by 4 weeks.

After that, if you feel ready, you can switch to the "Next Level" training program.

Estimated time

7 to 10 weeks for a concrete result.

The test gave you a result of more than 20%.

It will take at least 3 months to start seeing an aesthetic result because you have 9 kg and more to lose.

Above 10 kg of overweight, it is good to start further in stages.

You could also in this case, extend the preparatory program by one or two weeks, but I would advise you to choose a softer approach, evaluating a more suitable route for your starting situation.

In this regard, I suggest you consult my article/guide "Training to lose weight: the best strategies for success" (content in Italian).

Step 3: Workout Routines for beginner.

This 4-week preparation routine will familiarize you with the exercises and at the same time you will begin to understand my "philosophy", the rhythms of training and everything related to my method.

If you haven't trained or haven't followed a constant workout for more than a month, don't skip this step, believe me! You'll risk dropping everything.

It may seem strange to you to train with a few exercises that "apparently" train few muscles. Actually, I'm going to tell you something that's going to make you very angry.

Of all those myriad exercises with dumbbells, ankle braces and elastics, very few are aimed at a general and harmonious toning of YOUR body, talkless your abs.

By training the large muscle groups, you will indirectly train almost all small muscle groups, i.e. those you train with various curls, extensions etc. etc.

So, who specifically needs to train the biceps or the triceps?

The bodybuilder lacking the muscle and those who, already having a good physique, want to improve a small muscle (the example of the biceps).

But those who do not have a great physique and are already deficient in large muscle groups, it makes no sense for them to concentrate on the so-called isolation exercises.

Therefore, the large muscle groups that we are going to treat will be:

- Bibs

- Dorsals

- Quadriceps and Hips.

Focusing on the main exercises to stimulate these muscles will train indirectly (I will only mention the main ones):

- Triceps, biceps, shoulders, abdominals and lumbar.

So why do 10-12 exercises per session? That's just it, why?

Obviously the abdominals will also be trained in a special and direct way, on the other hand, your goal is to have a super toned abdomen!

In the following pages, you will find 2 simple tables describing the 2 training plans and pictures of the exercises. (routines at the gym, at home bodywheygt, at home with dumbbell, at home with dumbbell and bench, at home trx)

First, don't forget to warm up before each workout.

WEEKLY PREPARATORY TRAINING PROGRAMS FOR BEGINNERS (4 WEEKS.)

Gym Routine.

Number of workouts: 3/4 Weekly workouts *(Monday-Wednesday-Friday advice)*

Flat Bench Press	4x(20 sec. + 45 rec.)
Squat	4x(20 sec. + 45 rec.)
Chest Press	4x(20 sec. + 45 rec.)
Classic Crunch	4x(25 sec. + 45 rec.)
Reverse Crunch	4x(20 sec. + 45 rec.)

Bodyweight Routine

Number of workouts: ¾ Weekly workouts *(Monday-Wednesday-Friday advice)*

Push Ups	4x(20 sec. + 45 rec.)
Squat	4x(20 sec. + 45 rec.)
V – Push Ups	4x(20 sec. + 45 rec.)
Classic Crunch	4x(25 sec. + 45 rec.)
Reverse Crunch	4x(20 sec. + 45 rec.)

Routine with dumbbells.

Number of workouts: 3/4 Weekly workouts
(Monday-Wednesday-Friday advice)

Push Ups	4x(20 sec. + 45 rec.)
Squat	4x(20 sec. + 45 rec.)
Dumbbell Floor Press	4x(20 sec. + 45 rec.)
Classic Crunch	4x(25 sec. + 45 rec.)
Reverse Crunch	4x(20 sec. + 45 rec.)

Routine with dumbbells and bech.

Number of workouts: 3/4 Weekly workouts
(Monday-Wednesday-Friday advice)

Flat Bench Press	4x(20 sec. + 45 rec.)
Squat	4x(20 sec. + 45 rec.)
One-Arm Dumbbell Row	4x(20 sec. + 45 rec.)
Classic Crunch	4x(25 sec. + 45 rec.)
Reverse Crunch	4x(20 sec. + 45 rec.)

TRX Routine.

Number of workouts: 3/4 Weekly workouts
(Monday-Wednesday-Friday advice)

TRX Push Up	4x(20 sec. + 45 rec.)
Squat TRX	4x(20 sec. + 45 rec.)
Back Row TRX	4x(20 sec. + 45 rec.)
TRX sit up	4x(25 sec. + 45 rec.)
Reverse Crunch	4x(20 sec. + 45 rec.)

WEEKLY AEROBIC TRAINING PROGRAM

	WEEK 1	WEEK 2
Aerobic Training	2 or 3 *	2 or 3 *
Training IT	0 or 1*	0 or 1*

*evaluate based on your starting condition. If you have not done regular aerobic training in the last 2 weeks, start with IT only from the 2nd week.

INDICATIONS

All beginners training should be done 3 times a week and lasts about 25 minutes.

A total of 4 series of training sessions should be performed. Recovery between one series and the other.

As you can see, I have not entered a precise number of repetitions just to give you the opportunity to do the best you can do in a specific time frame.

For rec. It means simple recovery.

Aerobic Training

30 minutes.

You should be equipped with a heart rate monitor and during aerobic workouts, maintain a range of 65%-75% of your maximum frequency.

[formula: 208 man/211 woman - (age x 0.7)]. Do the aerobics you prefer! (running, biking, cycling, swimming, etc.)

Aerobic IT

We increase the intensity by entering the interval training (IT). What is it? A training in which you will alternate various rhythms of training:

- 5 minutes warm-up time

- 2' at medium/low intensity (65-75% f.max)

- 1' at medium/high intensity (75-85% f.max)

- Repeat the cycle 6 times

- 2 minutes light intensity cool down.

Step 4: Workout Routines Next Level

If you have had a look at the "Workout Routines for Beginner" section, you will need to structure an evolution of that program and follow it for 4 weeks.

IMPORTANT NOTE: "NO FAT" version: if you have less than 10% fat mass, recovery will ALWAYS be simple.

*for rec. This means simple recovery, while **R.A.** means "active recovery": you will have to do any aerobic activity that will increase your pulse rate so much (if you don't have equipment such as exercise bikes or tapis, you can think about jumping rope or running on the spot).

Are you enjoying this book? I really hope so! I would be really happy if you could leave a short Amazon review, I am very interested to know what you think. Thank you

Gym Routine.

Number of workouts: 3/4 Weekly workouts *(Monday-Wednesday-Friday advice)*

	WEEK 1	WEEK 2	WEEK 3	WEEK 4
Incline Bench Press	4x(20 sec. + 45 **R.A.****)	4x(25 sec. + 40 R.A.)	4x(25 sec. + 40 R.A.)	2x(25 sec. + 40 R.A.)
Squat Jump	4x(20 sec. + 45 R.A.)	4x(25 sec. + 40 R.A)	4x(25 sec. + 40 R.A)	2x(25 sec. + 40 R.A)
Chest Press	4x(20 sec. + 45 rec.)	4x(25 sec. + 40 rec.)	4x(30 sec. + 35 rec.)	2x(30 sec. + 35

				rec.)
Twist on Fitness Ball	4x(25 sec. + 45 R.A.)	4x(30 sec. + 40 R.A.)	4x(35 sec. + 35 R.A.)	2x(35 sec. + 35 R.A.)
Hollow Position	4x(25 sec. + 45 R.A.)	4x(30 sec. + 40 R.A.)	4x(35 sec. + 35 R.A.)	2x(35 sec. + 35 R.A.)

Bodyweight Routine

Number of workouts: 3/4 Weekly workouts *(Monday-Wednesday-Friday advice)*

	WEEK 1	WEEK 2	WEEK 3	WEEK 4
Push ups with feet	4x(20 sec. + 45	4x(25 sec. + 40	4x(25 sec. + 40	2x(25 sec. + 40

elevated	R.A.**)	R.A.)	R.A.)	R.A.)
Diamond Push ups	4x(20 sec. + 45 R.A.)	4x(25 sec. + 40 R.A)	4x(25 sec. + 40 R.A)	2x(25 sec. + 40 R.A)
Squat Jump	4x(20 sec. + 45 rec.)	4x(25 sec. + 40 rec.)	4x(30 sec. + 35 rec.)	2x(30 sec. + 35 rec.)
Twist on Fitness Ball	4x(25 sec. + 45 R.A.)	4x(30 sec. + 40 R.A.)	4x(35 sec. + 35 R.A.)	2x(35 sec. + 35 R.A.)
Hollow Position	4x(25 sec. + 45 R.A.)	4x(30 sec. + 40 R.A.)	4x(35 sec. + 35 R.A.)	2x(35 sec. + 35 R.A.)

Routine with dumbbells.

Number of workouts: 3/4 Weekly workouts
(Monday-Wednesday-Friday advice)

	WEEK 1	WEEK 2	WEEK 3	WEEK 4
Push ups with feet elevated	4x(20 sec. + 45 **R.A.****)	4x(25 sec. + 40 R.A.)	4x(25 sec. + 40 R.A.)	2x(25 sec. + 40 R.A.)
One Arm Dumbbell Floor Press	4x(20 sec. + 45 R.A.)	4x(25 sec. + 40 R.A)	4x(25 sec. + 40 R.A)	2x(25 sec. + 40 R.A)
Squat Jump	4x(20 sec. + 45 rec.)	4x(25 sec. + 40 rec.)	4x(30 sec. + 35 rec.)	2x(30 sec. + 35 rec.)
Twist on Fitness Ball	4x(25 sec. + 45 R.A.)	4x(30 sec. + 40 R.A.)	4x(35 sec. + 35 R.A.)	2x(35 sec. + 35 R.A.)

Hollow Position	4x(25 sec. + 45 R.A.)	4x(30 sec. + 40 R.A.)	4x(35 sec. + 35 R.A.)	2x(35 sec. + 35 R.A.)

Routine with dumbbells and bech.

Number of workouts: 3/4 Weekly workouts *(Monday-Wednesday-Friday advice)*

	WEEK 1	WEEK 2	WEEK 3	WEEK 4
Incline Bench Press	4x(20 sec. + 45 **R.A.****)	4x(25 sec. + 40 R.A.)	4x(25 sec. + 40 R.A.)	2x(25 sec. + 40 R.A.)
One Arm Dumbbell Floor Press	4x(20 sec. + 45 R.A.)	4x(25 sec. + 40 R.A)	4x(25 sec. + 40 R.A)	2x(25 sec. + 40 R.A)
Squat Jump	4x(20 sec. + 45 rec.)	4x(25 sec. + 40 rec.)	4x(30 sec. + 35 rec.)	2x(30 sec. + 35 rec.)

Twist on Fitness Ball	4x(25 sec. + 45 R.A.)	4x(30 sec. + 40 R.A.)	4x(35 sec. + 35 R.A.)	2x(35 sec. + 35 R.A.)
Hollow Position	4x(25 sec. + 45 R.A.)	4x(30 sec. + 40 R.A.)	4x(35 sec. + 35 R.A.)	2x(35 sec. + 35 R.A.)

TRX Routine.

Number of workouts: 3/4 Weekly workouts *(Monday-Wednesday-Friday advice)*

	WEEK 1	WEEK 2	WEEK 3	WEEK 4
TRX Push Ups	4x(20 sec. + 45 **R.A.****)	4x(25 sec. + 40 R.A.)	4x(25 sec. + 40 R.A.)	2x(25 sec. + 40 R.A.)
Squat Jump	4x(20 sec. +	4x(25 sec. +	4x(25 sec. +	2x(25 sec. +

TRX	45 R.A.)	40 R.A)	40 R.A)	40 R.A)
TRX Chest Fly	4x(20 sec. + 45 rec.)	4x(25 sec. + 40 rec.)	4x(30 sec. + 35 rec.)	2x(30 sec. + 35 rec.)
TRX Crunch	4x(25 sec. + 45 R.A.)	4x(30 sec. + 40 R.A.)	4x(35 sec. + 35 R.A.)	2x(35 sec. + 35 R.A.)
TRX Pike	4x(25 sec. + 45 R.A.)	4x(30 sec. + 40 R.A.)	4x(35 sec. + 35 R.A.)	2x(35 sec. + 35 R.A.)

WEEKLY AEROBIC TRAINING PROGRAM

	WEEK 1	WEEK 2	WEEK 3	WEEK 4
Aerobic Training	1	1	1	1
Training IT	2	2	1	0
HIIT Training	0	0	1	2

INDICATIONS

Free body training should be done 3 times a week and lasts about 25 minutes.

I know you want sculpted abs, but believe me, you can't tone your abdomen and walk around with arms and pecs NOT up to the mark.

Also, training these muscle groups, in addition to squatting your legs, will help you further increase your metabolism and make your body a real fat-burning furnace!

So, follow the pattern to the letter and trust what I tell you

For the first 3 weeks, perform a total of 4 series of exercise with a total recovery time between each series.

As you can see, I didn't enter a precise number of repetitions just to give you the chance to do the best you can do in a precise time frame.

Study the table well in order not to miss the differences (sometimes minimal) between one week and another.

Rec. means simple recovery, while R.A. means "active recovery":

You'll have to do any aerobic activity that will increase your pulse rate so much (if you don't have equipment like exercise bikes or tapis, you can think about jumping rope or running on the spot).

During week 4, the exhaust week, you only do 2 series.

Aerobic Training

40 minutes.

You should be equipped with a heart rate monitor and during aerobic workouts, keep within a range of 65%-75% of your maximum frequency [formula: 208man/211woman - (age x 0.7)]. Do the aerobic activity you prefer! (running, biking, cycling, swimming, etc.)

Aerobic IT

We increase the intensity by entering the interval training (IT). What is it? A workout in which you will alternate various training rhythms:

- 5 minutes warm-up time

- 2 minutes at medium/low intensity (65-75% f.max)

- 1 minute at medium-high intensity (75-85% f.max)

- Repeat the cycle 6 times

- 2 minutes cool down.

HIIT:

You can run outdoors or on the treadmill by

adjusting your heart rate (same for the exercise bike or bicycle).

1. 3' pulse heating 55%-65% f.max

2. 1' pulse 65-75% f.max.

3. 1' pulsation 75-85% f.max

4. 1' pulse 85-90% f.max

5. 1' fast walk or very slow recovery run.

6. Points 2-3-4-5 must be repeated 5 times in all.

7. 2-minutes cool down.

EXERCISE DESCRIPTION (PHOTO)

Flat Bench Press

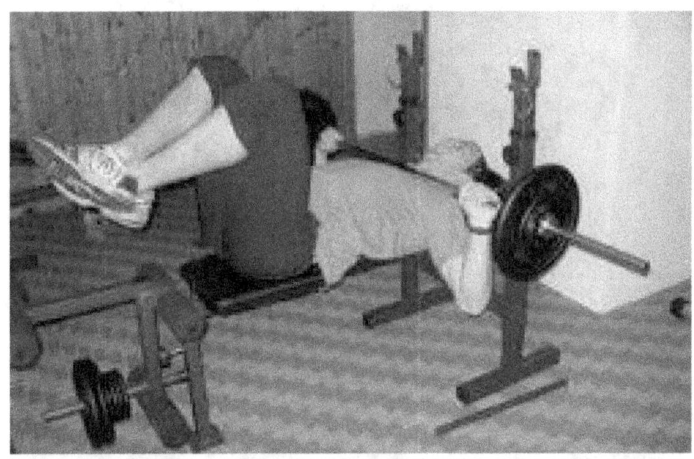

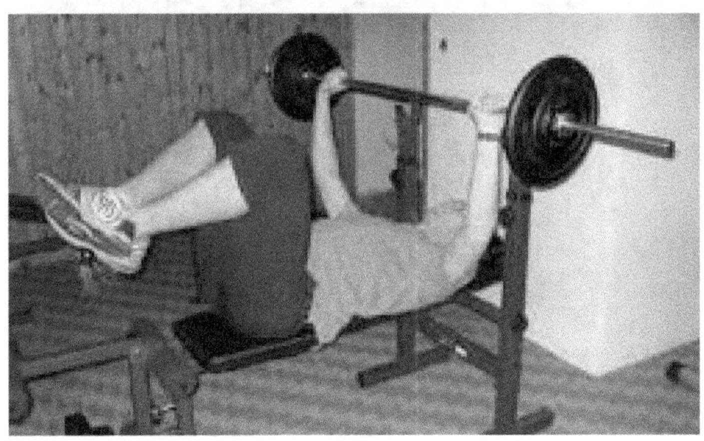

Incline Bench Press

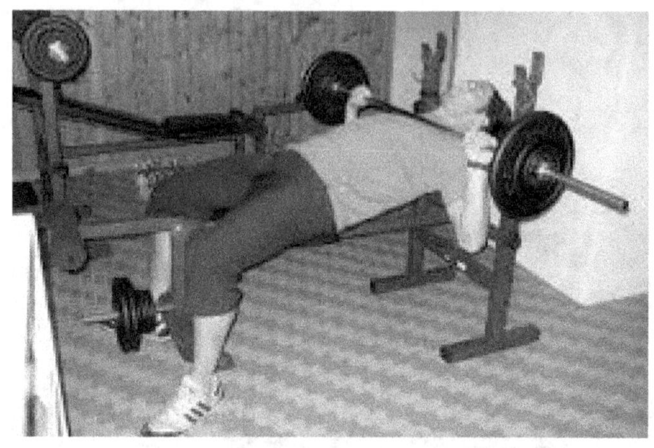

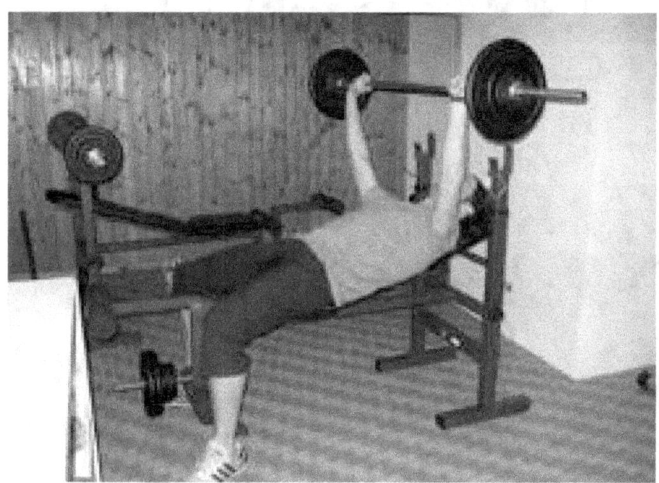

Push Ups

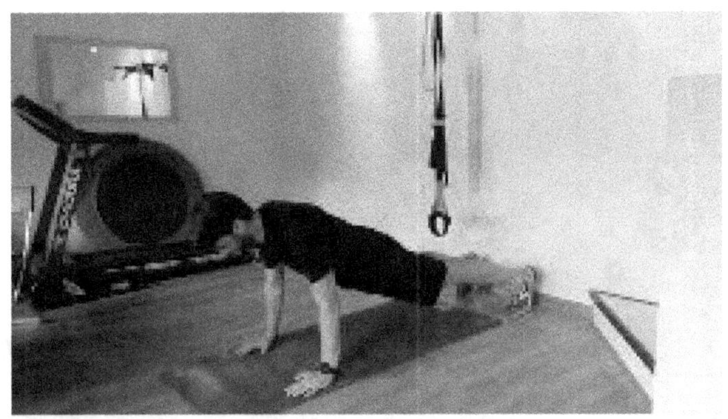

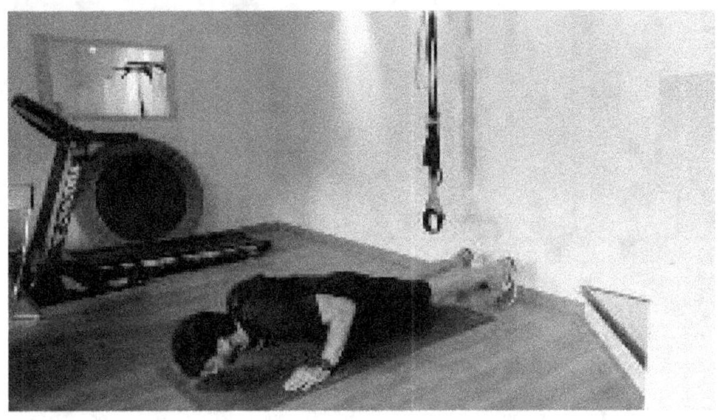

V-Push Ups

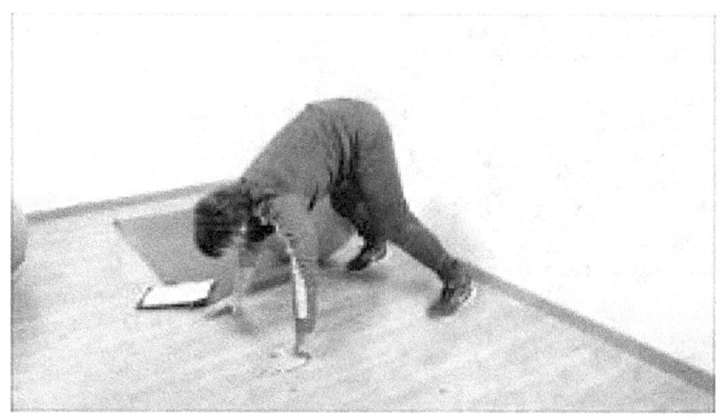

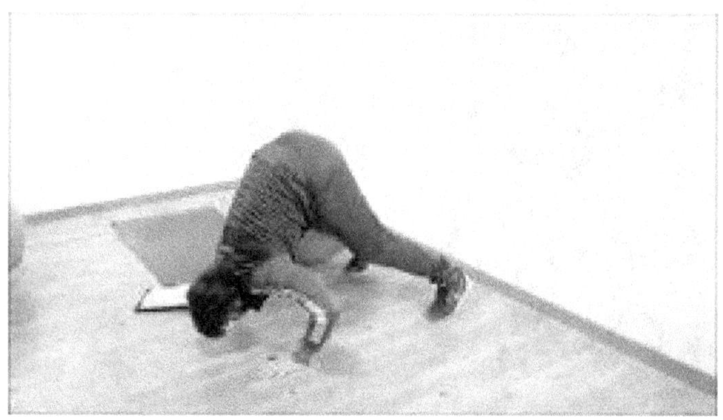

TRX Push Up

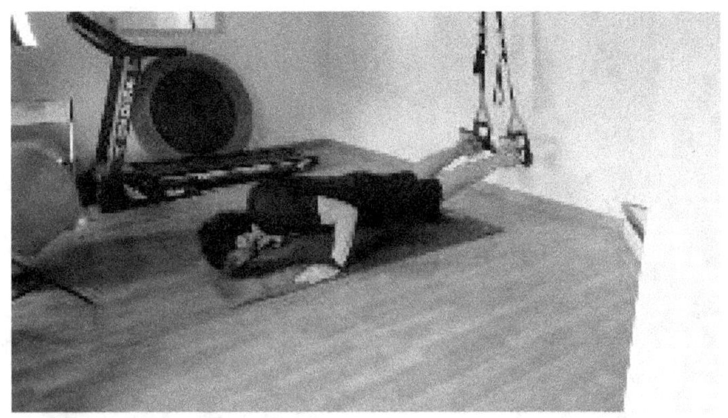

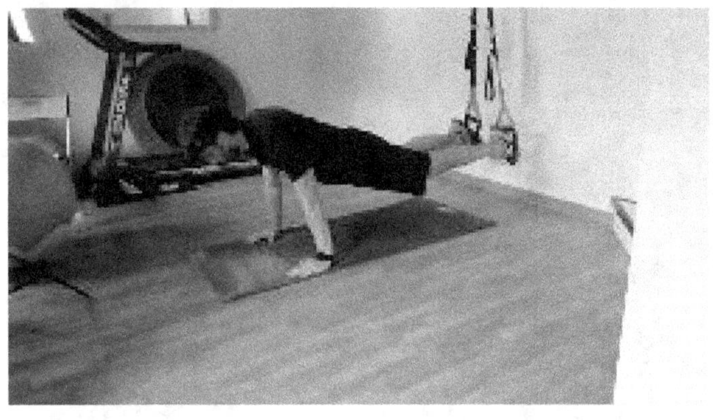

Diamond Push ups

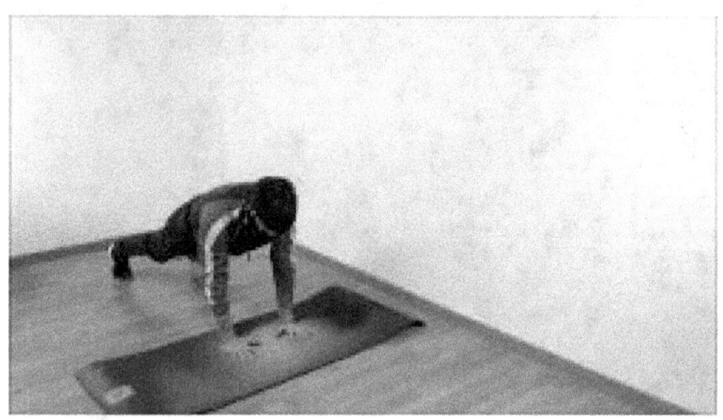

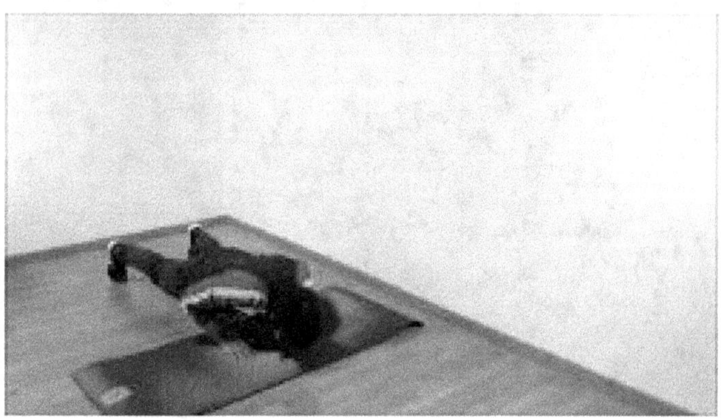

Push ups with feet elevated

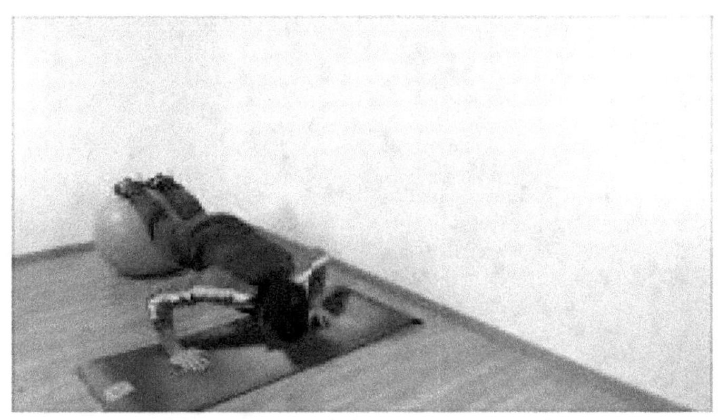

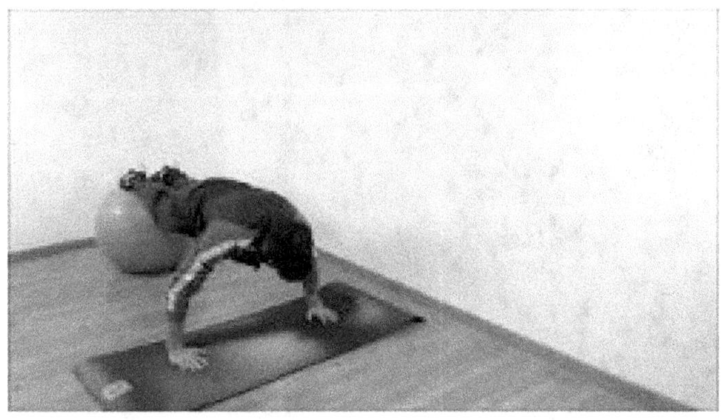

Dumbbell Floor Press

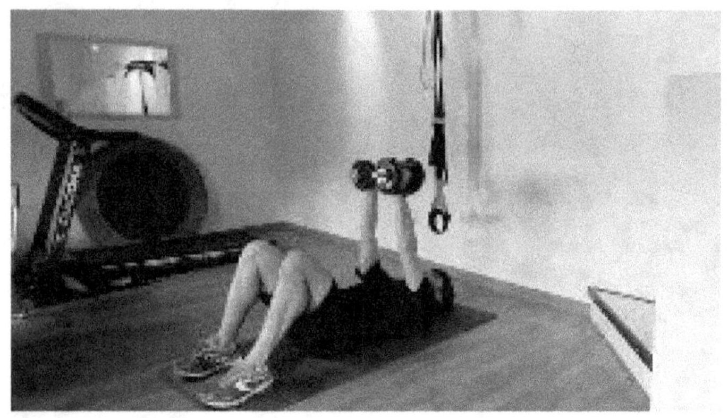

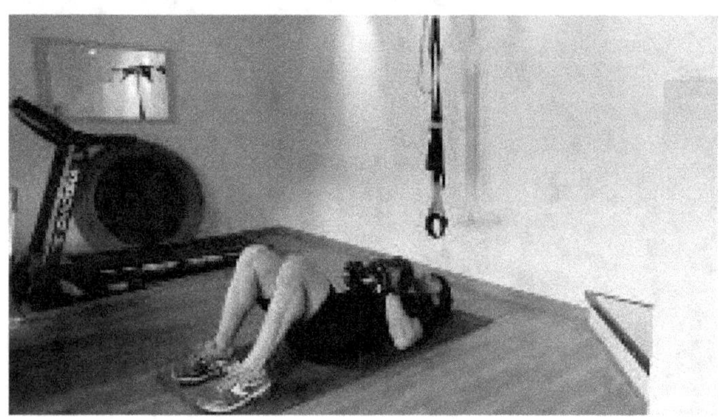

One Arm Dumbbell Floor Press

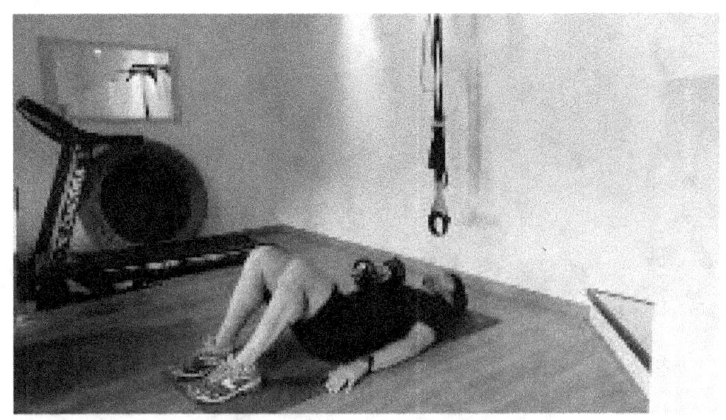

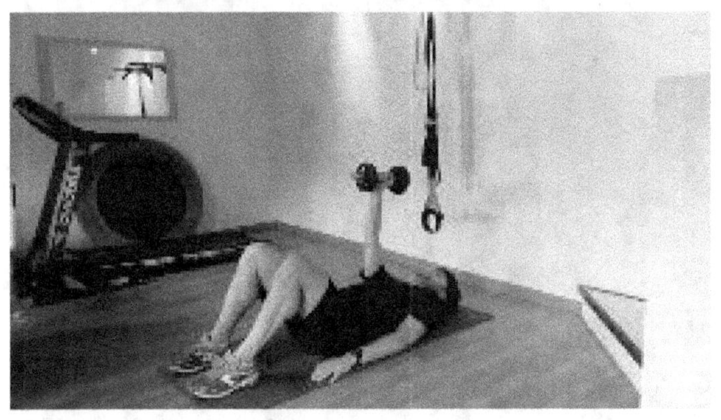

Chest Press

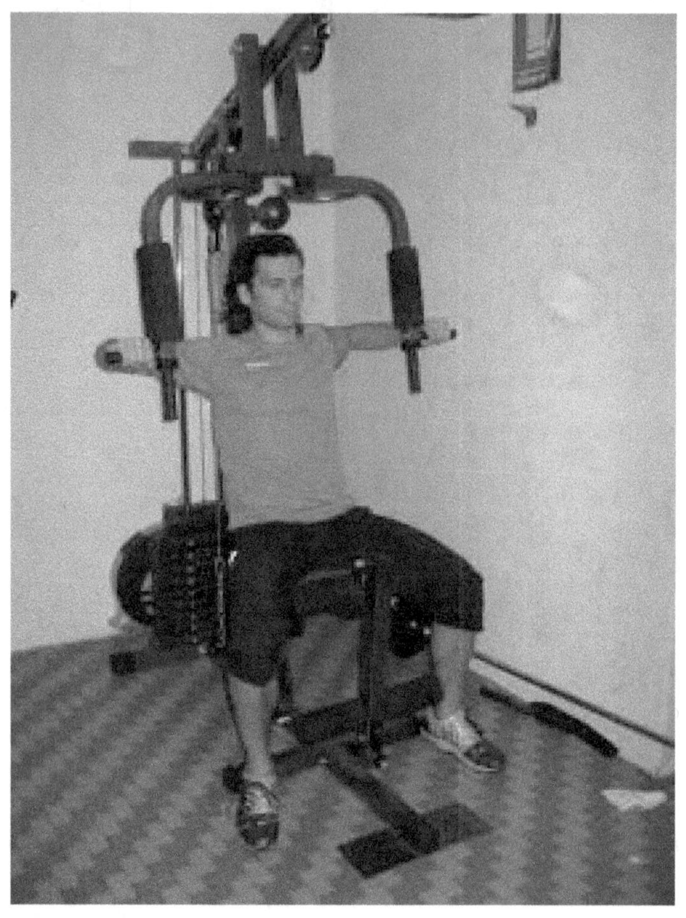

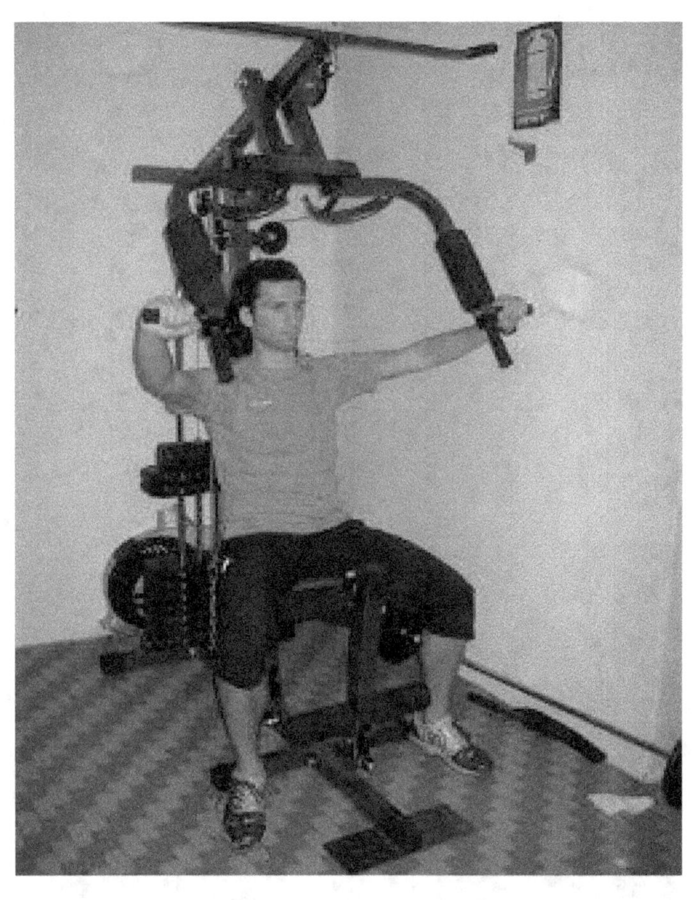

TRX Chest Fly

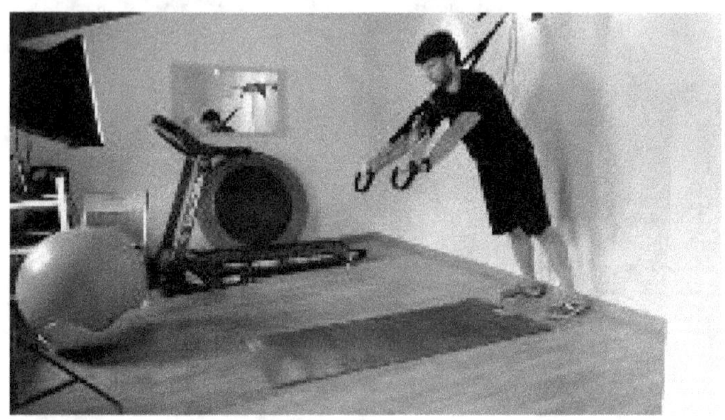

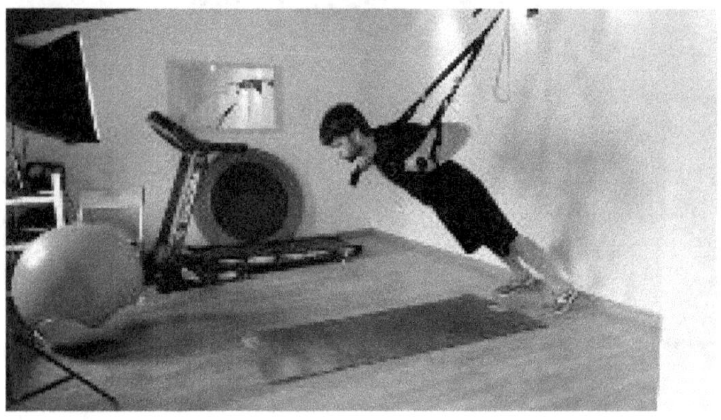

66

One-Arm Dumbbell Row

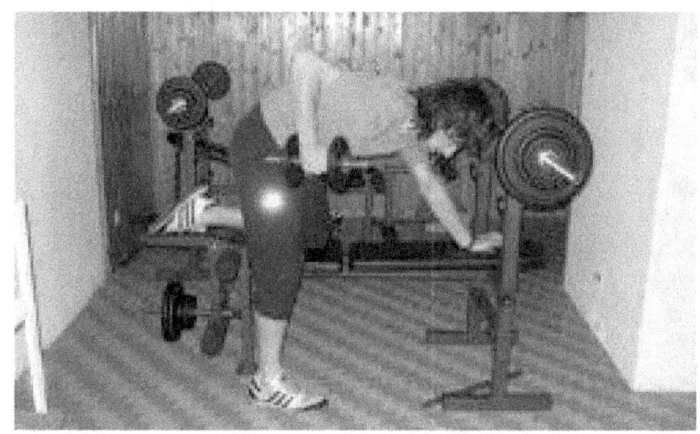

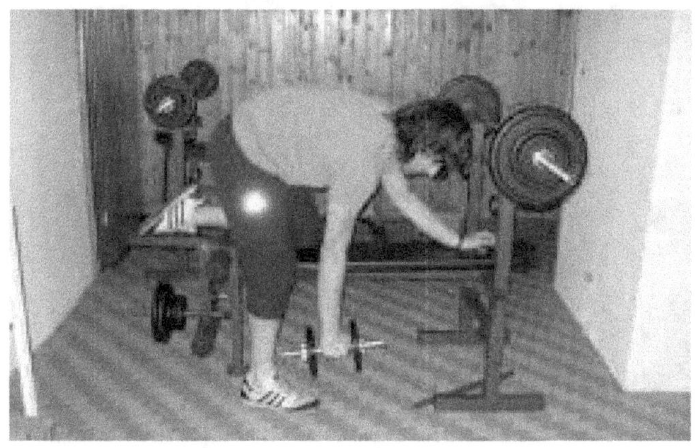

Back Row TRX

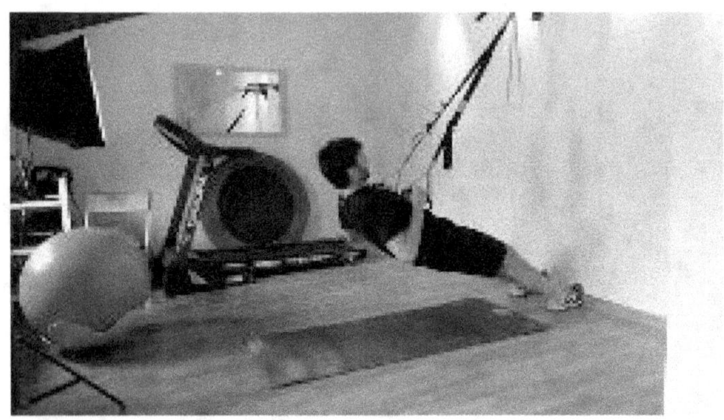

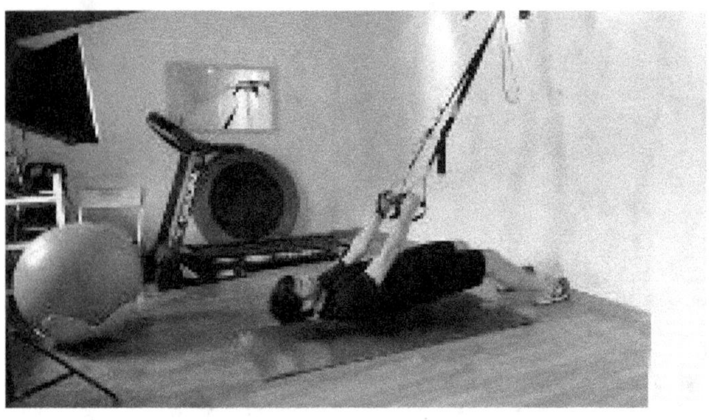

Squat

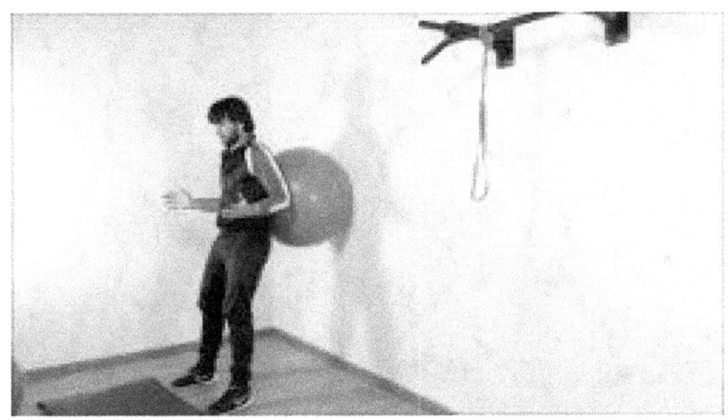

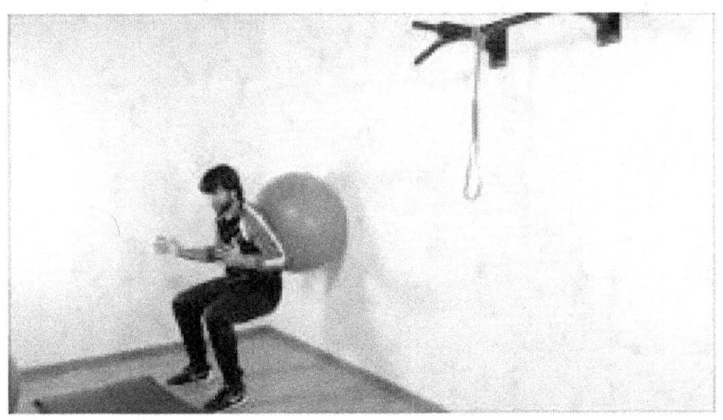

Squat TRX

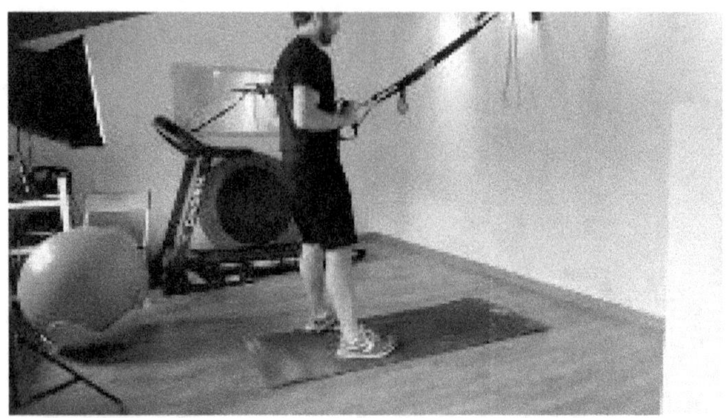

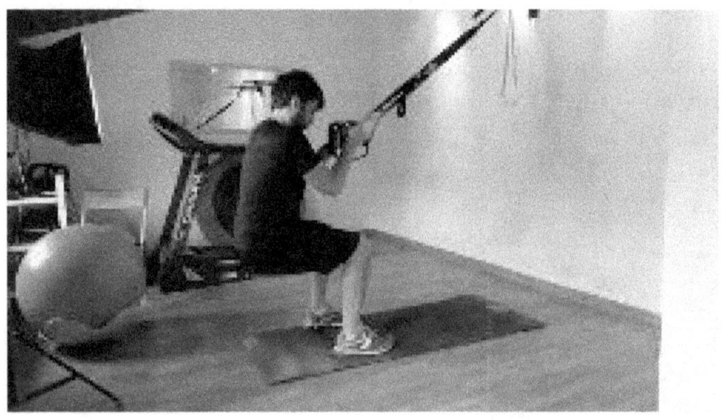

Squat Jump

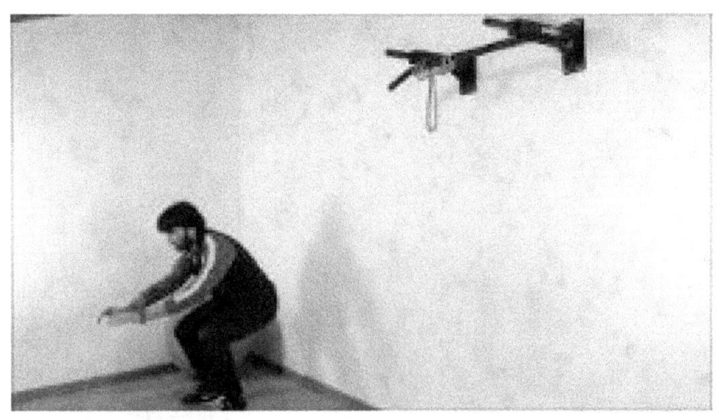

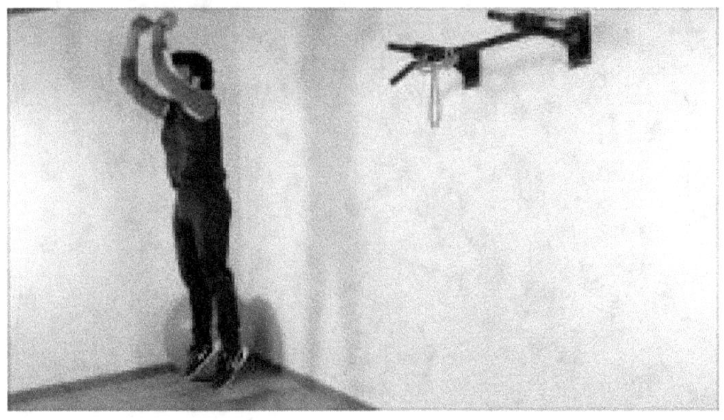

Squat Jump TRX

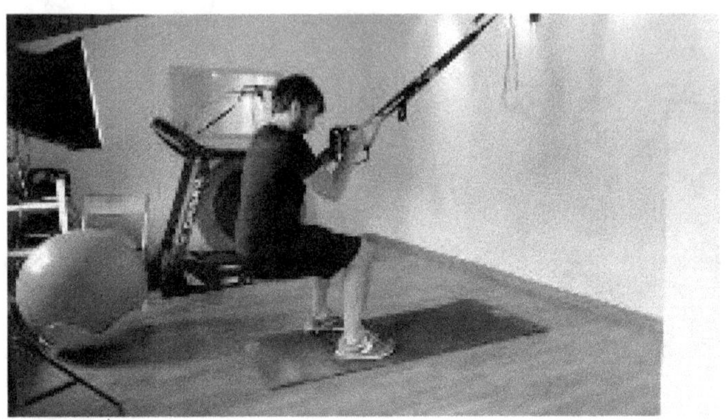

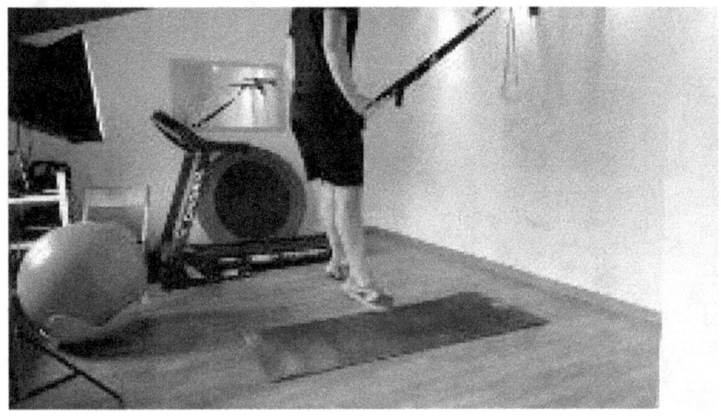

Classic Crunch

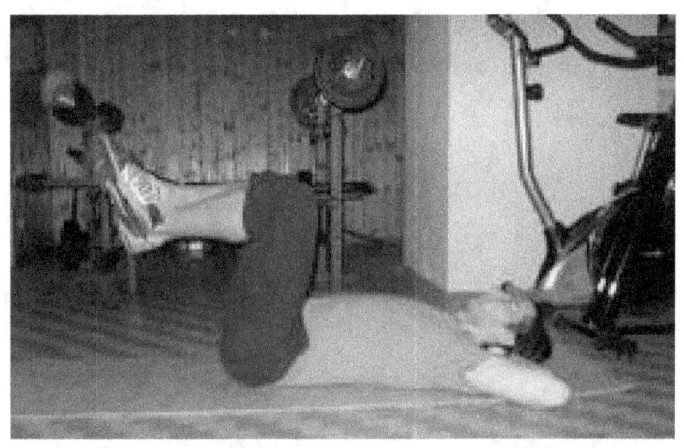

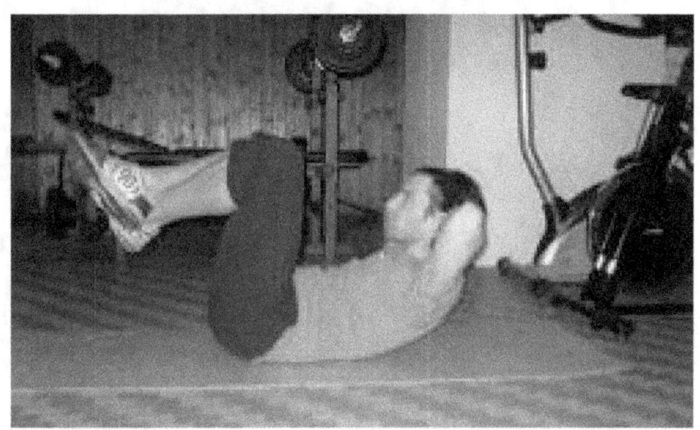

Reverse Crunch

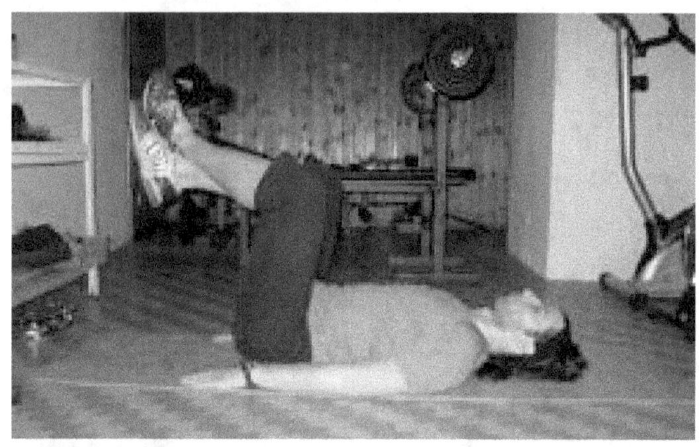

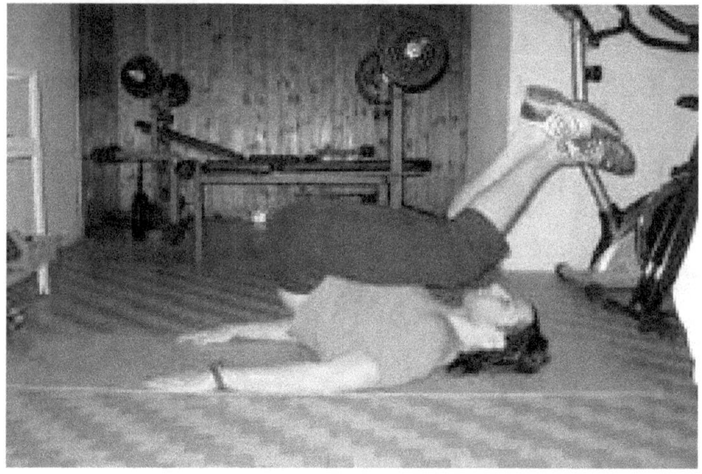

74

Hollow Position

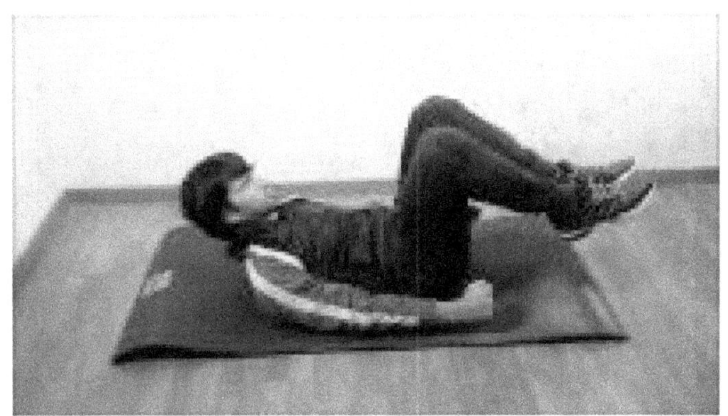

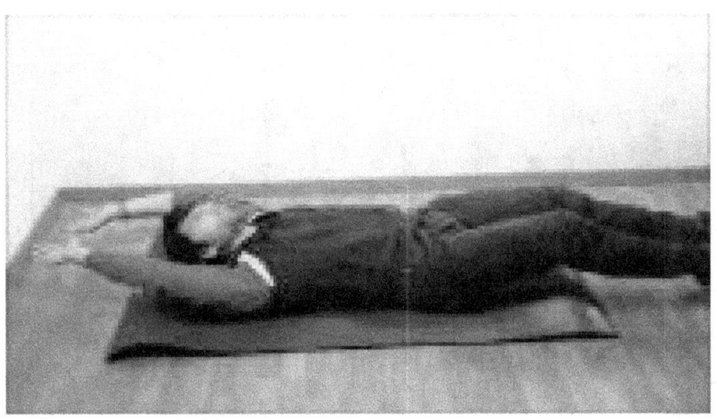

75

TRX sit up

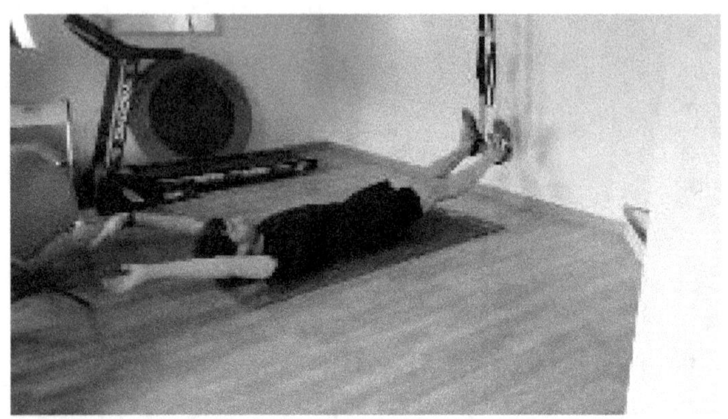

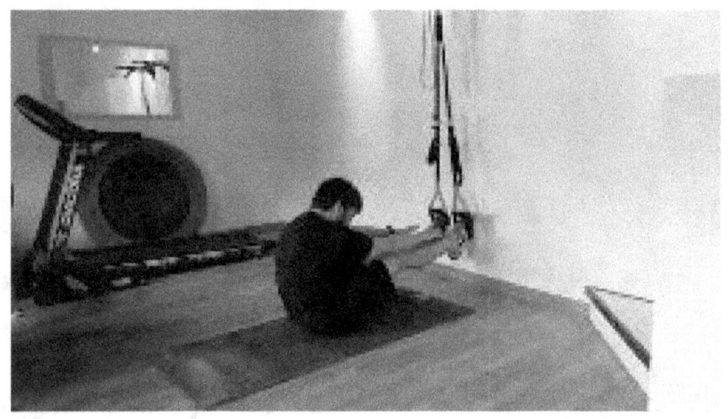

Twist on Fitness Ball

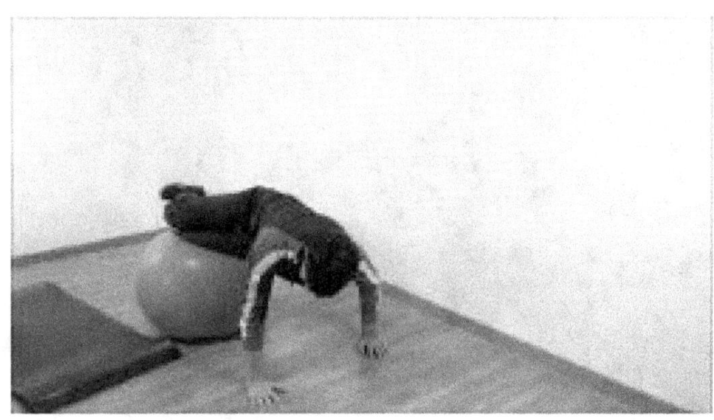

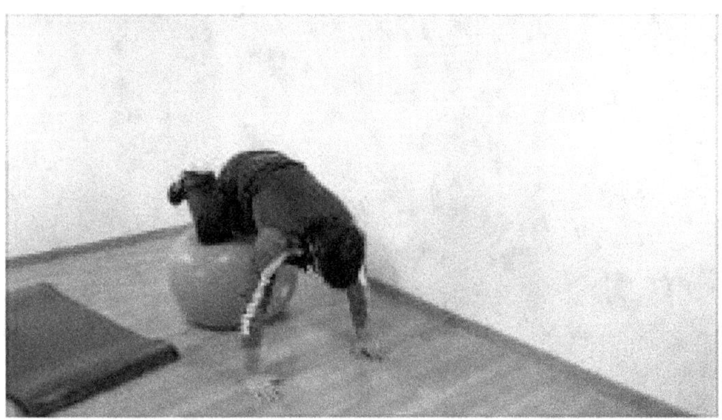

TRX Crunch

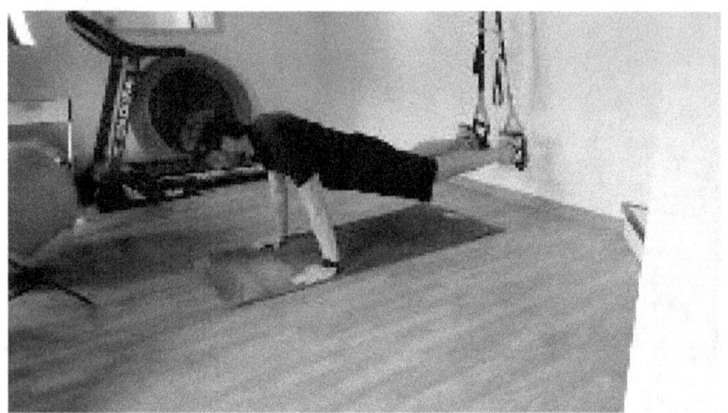

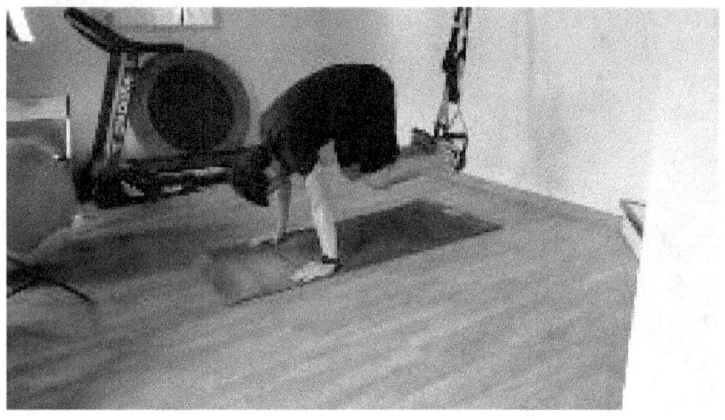

TRX Pike

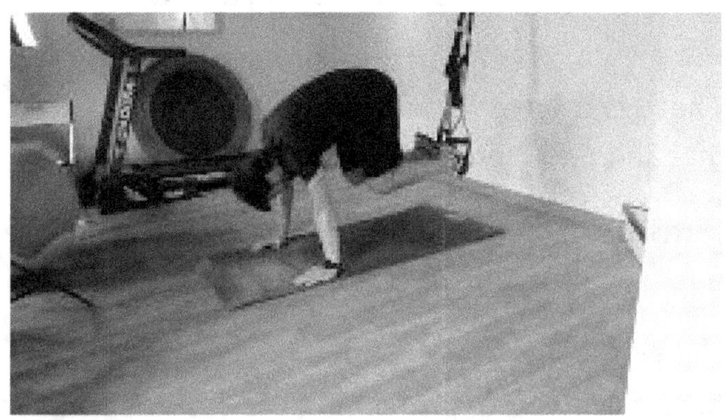

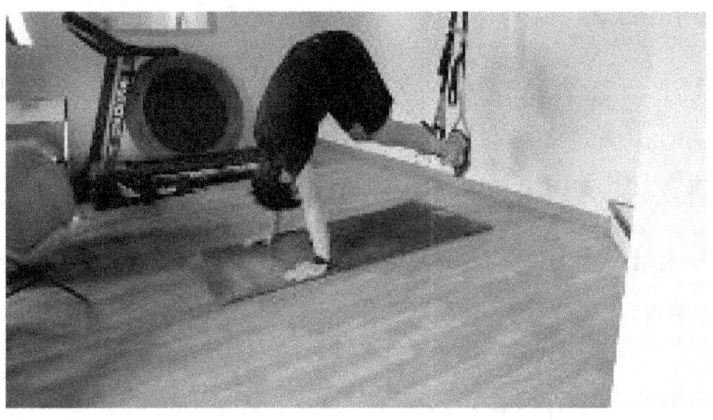

PURIFY YOUR BODY AND LEARN TO FEED CLEANLY.

There is a lot of confusion about the concept of diet and nutrition.

Nutrition is not a pleasure. It is, indeed the case but for our organism, it represents vital energy.

Unfortunately, if we indulge ourselves too much, food becomes a problem, in the sense that it makes us fat!

This often leads us to " fight" with food and consider it a tempting enemy that makes us regret having eaten it.

In this chapter, I want to teach you how to make peace with food, starting with "Metabolism", how to understand it and then " trick" it so that we can eat in freedom!

We can define metabolism as the set of all the processes that lead the body to transform the food we ingest into ready-to-use energy.

It is by no means an organ, that must be clear to you. Let's see how it works.

Metabolism can act in 2 ways: catabolism and anabolism.

The first uses energy to destroy cells (muscle or fat) while the second allows the body to use energy to "build" your body.

So, it will be easy for you to guess, if you don't have enough energy, your body won't perform the catabolism process in the optimal way and as a result, you will have less fat loss, which if it covers your belly, will prevent you from seeing your abs.

Moreover, if you eat too little or too badly, it won't even trigger muscle anabolism! I remind you that, the more muscle you have, the more your body burns to sustain itself.

To sum up and make you understand better, if you don't provide all the nutrients...:

- Fat catabolism is not triggered correctly

- You won't gain muscle because anabolism will suffer.

- With less muscle, your metabolism will be slow and therefore consume much less.

All this necessary preamble is to make you understand what I'm about to tell you. To make your life easier (and reading it) I'm going to make it easy for you with a bulleted list:

- You have to consider food as an essential source to achieve your optimal shape.

- You have to eat to lose weight! If you don't eat, you won't lose weight! You lose weight because you lose muscles.

- The amount of food you eat is much less important than the quality of the food you eat.

- Eating 2 ounces of lean meat is not the same as eating 2 ounces of French fries! The quantity is the same, but the calorie intake is very different, as meat brings nutrients to your body, while chips bring a lot of heavy fat typical of fries.

On that last point, I want you to focus your attention.

Taking the example, the potato would not be a harmful or discarded food. The problem lies in the way it is cooked. Frying greatly increases the calories and also enriches the food with fat.

So, you can easily understand that those calories are "free" calories, that is, they don't serve to give you satiety, they just serve to take you easily beyond your needs and as you know, excess calories = accumulated fat.

With this, I don't want to say that you have to ban fried foods, sweets or particularly seasoned and elaborated foods (on the contrary, later on, we will see how junk food meals are fundamental for the success of the diet), but only that in our diet, we have to focus on healthy and tasty foods that allow us to eat to satiation and give the body everything it needs.

For this reason, I will now give you a small list of "ok" foods and those that belong to the category "to limit":

- Vegetables. I'll be brief. Vegetables are a must. Few calories compared to a good intake of useful carbohydrates and vitamins.

- Legumes. Same thing for legumes and in addition, they provide vegetable proteins, useful to fill the total need of proteins.

- Meat. Meat is a fundamental food.

Essential for the health of the body, in fact, it guarantees the number of proteins needed. They are an "ok" food, with preference for white meat (chicken, turkey, etc...).

- Fish. Another perfectly "ok" food! Noble proteins and enzymes essential for the body's processes.

- Pasta. Pasta is another food that can be part of our diet. You can eat it every day, even though I prefer 3-4 times a week and preferably at lunchtime. Always remember to keep an eye on the seasonings.

- Bread and other baked goods. Bread can be considered "ok" by limiting its consumption. For example, a small portion at lunch like a small sandwich. More elaborate products such as pizzas and focaccia are "to be limited" because they contain many calories and too many empty carbohydrates (useless if not fattened if not burned immediately).

- Cheese and salami. They would be "to limit", but I have always eaten them regularly at practically every dinner. Watch out, however, to the quantities (3 slices of ham and 30 grams of cheese is already almost too much) and as a sausage, raw ham is preferable, and salami is forbidden.

- Sweets. In the morning at breakfast, you can eat biscuits, cookies, and some not too elaborate desserts. Cakes and pastries should be limited as much as possible. I recommend only on special occasions, otherwise max once a week.

Fruit. All types of fruit are good because they contain a lot of vitamins and substances essential for the regular functioning of our body. Be careful not to overdo it. Fruit contains a lot of simple sugars, so large amounts of fruit would make you fat!

Seasonings. I firmly believe that they are the big problem for those who want sculpted abs (along with beer and other spirits .) Always be careful how much and what seasoning you use.

The oil is often used to grease the pan so that the food does not "stick". Whether or not it's a good system, I don't see why I should increase the caloric intake of the food out of all foods, including vegetables. Same goes for butter.

A good Diet for Weight Loss does not exclude oil, but limits its raw consumption. Cooking oil can increase calorie intake by up to 10 times! Eliminating it, I can afford much more generous portions, providing useful nutrients to the body and not harmful and rich in fat, as can be the cooked oil.

The first thing to do in order to find your balance will be to insert one day a week in which, with criterion, you can enjoy your gluttony and get out of order with "forbidden condiments" and / or junk food.

In addition to the day off, another thing that should never be missing is the mid-morning and mid-afternoon snack. This is because, digestion still requires caloric consumption, just as if it were an activity you do. In fact, calories are spent both during digestion and assimilation of your meals (thermal effect of food)..

So, the more you eat during the day, the more calories you consume...

The thermal effect consumes about 10% of the

total calories you spend every day. Protein has the highest thermal effect, followed by carbohydrates and fats last.

That's why, eating a small portion of lean protein at every meal is a great way to burn more calories. It also helps to limit your blood sugar levels and give you a sense of satiety.

Every time you have a meal, you spend calories in the digestive process and absorption of the meal. So if you eat 5/6 small meals during the day, instead of 2/3 heavy meals, all you do is increase your calorie consumption by simply eating several times.

In addition, you should know that the stomach is very "elastic" and has the ability to adapt to the amount of food ingested. When you eat 3 heavy meals, your stomach expands to contain all the food you eat in a single session.

To make you better understand the concept: after eating a large meal, go in front of the mirror and take a look at your stomach. It's huge.

On the contrary, if you eat 5/6 small meals, your stomach doesn't strain to swell to contain a large volume of food. And in this case, if you looked in the mirror, you would notice that your stomach is smaller than the previous case.

This is a simple and effective trick that many models and personal trainers use to maintain an enviable shape!

How to Act

After so much theory, I will now show you what to do in practice, with examples on how to set your "food day".

Here is how to act:

- Cleanse yourself.

- Hydrate.

- Adjust.

- Plan.

Step 1: Cleanse yourself.

Food, especially junk food, produces toxins that prevent the body, among other things, from losing weight easily.

If you follow an unregulated diet and eat a lot of fried, overcooked, sweets and alcohol, then with the outline that we will see soon, you will get rid of many toxins and water retention, but you should follow a simple protocol of hydration and purification to get the best possible result.

I use some purifying herbal teas associated with lemon...

Step 2: Hydrate.

Hydration can easily be linked to purification, as it helps the body to get rid of toxins as well as excess fluids (water retention).

The classic advice of drinking at least 2 litres of water a day is a bit vague and does not take into account the differences from body to body.

However, as I do not have more precise parameters, I have successfully followed a personal protocol that allowed me to lose a lot of excess fluids in just 4 days.

Hydration is one of the most important things to be in shape.

The next chapter will be devoted entirely to hydration.

Step 3: Adjust.

- What foods to eat once a week.

    o Examples: Fries, very elaborate dishes, desserts, ice cream, beer, mayonnaise type sauces, sauces, heavy seasonings etc....

- What we can always eat in quantity.

    o vegetables, white meat, fish, etc.....

- What we can always eat but in moderation.

    o Fruit, dried fruit, vegetables, legumes, milk and dairy products etc.....

- What condiments to avoid and what we can always choose.

    o Avoid: cooking oil or butter and cream.

FAVORITE: all types of spices and sauces based on yoghurt.

Step 4: Plan

I'll say that, you won't have to go out of your mind and create a special menu, but for me, it was very important to create a weekly schedule in which I wrote down the type of food I was going to eat at each meal. This is also useful for shopping.

This suggestion is especially useful to avoid improvising.

Step 5: How do I feed myself for carved abs.

I would like to say that, this is NOT an indication of diet, but only a prospectus in which I describe the guidelines that are not the result of my "fantasy" but follow the instructions for a correct dietary education.

Breakfast

Your body hasn't hydrated for hours, so it may be a good idea to drink a cup of tea (or other "neutral" drink) with maybe half a lemon squeezed at breakfast.

Okay, now you have to eat. Yes, breakfast is not just coffee...

I usually eat some whole-grain biscuits with milk, but you can choose something else, for example cereal or toast. The important thing is to stick to common sense and don't always opt for croissants (once a week to treat yourself).

Mid-morning snack

Stay hydrated with a cup of purifying herbal tea and opt for a seasonal fruit.

Lunch

Here too, to make sure I'm hydrated enough, I drink two glasses of water first.

Keep filling up with half a portion of pasta or a loaf of bread by combining it with a source of protein, such as white meat or fish (minimum portion.) Accompany everything with plenty of vegetables or legumes.

Mid-afternoon snack

A cup of draining herbal tea and an unsweetened yogurt.

Dinner

The usual 2 glasses full of water first.

Give a stop to carbohydrates, the so called "empty" (bread and other baked goods) and opt for red meat (a couple of times a week) or white meat, fish (normal portion.) Always serve with vegetables or legumes.

Pre-sleep snack

A cup of relaxing herbal tea (chamomile tea) and a small source of protein (sliced lean or even half a glass of milk).

Post-workout snack (about 30 minutes)

Two glasses of water and a small source of protein (tuna or lean sliced meat).

HOW TO STAY HYDRATED

We've all heard the fact that our bodies are comprised of roughly 60% water. However, dehydration is incredibly common amongst those who exercise at *any* level. Many people do not know when they are dehydrated simply because they are not aware of the signs and symptoms. It is not unusual for both novice and avid athletes to neglect their hydration and later face the consequences.

Water, apart from oxygen, is the single most important thing we put into our bodies, and it should be treated as such. Whether you exercise every day or once a week, you need to be educated on the dangers of dehydration, the importance of staying hydrated, and how to hydrate properly.

The Dangers of Dehydration

We all know that regular exercise is an integral part of maintaining a healthy lifestyle. However, if you participate in any physical activity without ever taking in fluids, you are probably doing more harm than good. Chances are, you've been dehydrated at some point in time.

We lose water at an accelerated speed when we exercise our bodies. Sweating, for example, is a clear sign that your body is losing water. Losing fluids doesn't just mean losing water; it means losing all the electrolytes and minerals that the water carries, too. When we continue to lose fluids without replenishing them, we get dehydrated.

Dehydration of any degree can usually be felt right away. You may feel tired or weak; like your limbs are heavier than usual. Dehydration also contributes to muscle cramps and spasms, as well as headaches, light sensitivity, constipation, dry mouth and skin, and even dizziness.

Don't ever brush these symptoms off- especially if they come on suddenly. Water may be all that you're missing. If untreated, these symptoms will lead to reduced performance and subsequent reduced caloric burn and muscle gain. Whatever your goal is with your exercise, neglecting to hydrate is going to make it much, much harder to reach.

Unfortunately, one sip of water won't always cure you of dehydration. There is also such a thing as *long term* dehydration. This degree of dehydration can lead to severe headaches, high blood pressure, digestive disorders, back pain, kidney problems, and even heart disease.

Your organs need water to perform their tasks. Water helps circulate so many elements throughout your body. Blood, for example, carries proteins, lipids, minerals, and more to your muscles and organs. Without water, your blood cannot properly do its job. If you want your body to work properly, you *need* to give it what it needs.

It is incredibly important to stay hydrated during workouts, but it is something you should do all the time. It's okay if you forget your water bottle one day. But make sure it does not become a recurring incident.

How to Properly Hydrate

If you've been chugging a water bottle only once you're done your workout, you've been hydrating wrong. You need to take in fluids *before, during, and after* any physical activity (as well as on days when you aren't exercising, too). This will ensure you don't even get close to losing large amounts of fluids.

The amount of water you drink will depend on a number of factors, such as the intensity of the workout and environment (hot and humid versus cold, etc.). If you are unsure of how much water you should be drinking, divide your body weight (lbs) in half.

That is the amount of water (oz) you should be consuming *every single day*. Keep in mind, that is the amount of water you should be drinking on an *average* day.

As we now know, sweating during exercise means loss of fluids. So increase your average fluid intake accordingly. All you need is a 2-liter water bottle with you (slightly cool water is best), and you're good to go.

Make sure you take small sips throughout your physical activity. If your sport or exercise can allow it, try to take a small drink every 15 to 20 minutes. This will suffice if your exercise does not last more than 1 full hour. However, if your physical effort is needed for more than 1 hour, you will need to drink something other than water.

There are plenty of drinks on the market that have carbohydrates, electrolytes, and sodium. All of these minerals are lost during extensive workouts. Make sure you select a drink (other than water) that will replenish what you lost.

Sports drinks such as Gatorade (which contains sugars and potassium) are a very accessible option. If sports drinks aren't for you, there are plenty of other drinks you can make at home before heading out.

Cucumber and lemongrass water is a great (and tasty) way to add some flavor to your fluid intake. The combination of lemon, lime, and mint is another easy way to make hydrating a little more exciting. You can quickly make these drinks the night before a big workout, so they're ready to go in the morning.

Add in a few ice cubes to keep you cool. Don't think that hydrating needs to be boring and tasteless. The combinations are endless; all it takes is a sustained effort. Trust that it will get easier as you go on.

Believe it or not, the drinking you do *after* the workout is probably the most important. This is the time when you will do most of your rehydrating. Ideally, you should replace 150% of the fluids you lost. It is recommended you drink 1.5 liters of fluids per kilogram of weight lost.

The more you drink, the easier it will be to make it a habit. Drinking water shouldn't happen only when you feel thirsty. Oftentimes, dehydration builds up slowly over time. Make sure you drink at various points throughout the day. Start off with a small goal, like finishing one bottle every day. Then slowly build your way up. Your body will thank you for it- whether you're at the gym or not.

RECIPES FOR WEIGHT LOSS AND MUSCLE GAIN

Some people argue that you can only lose weight *or* gain muscle and never both at once. The truth is, losing excess fat while also putting on muscle is very much possible. All it takes is eating the right food and performing the right exercises at the right times.

Many people believe that in order to lose weight, you need to lower your consumption of food. But it's not always about *how much* you eat, but *what* you eat. Continue reading for some easy recipes that will help you not only lose the fat, but put on muscle too.

Spicy Tuna with Sweet Potato

This recipe is a delicious way to increase your protein intake, while remaining healthy and nutritious. This quick meal will provide you with 33 grams of protein and less than 1.8 grams of fat. Here's what you'll need:

For the tuna:

- 2 150g tuna steaks

- 1 tsp coarse sea salt

- 2 tbsp pink peppercorns

- 1 tbsp 100% melted coconut oil

For the sweet potato:

- 2 large sweet potatoes

- 1/2 tsp pepper

- 1/2 tsp salt

- 1 tbsp plain flour

- 1/2 tbsp melted coconut oil

Directions:

1. Preheat your oven to 200°C or 392 F

2. Clean your potatoes, poke holes in them with a fork, microwave them for 4 minutes

3. Once they have cooled, cut them into wedges. Drizzle coconut oil, flour, salt, and pepper over them. Feel free to add any spices you wish. Place them on a baking tray and bake them for 15-20 minutes.

4. Use this time to prepare your tuna steaks. Again, coat each steak with coconut oil and salt. Make sure you get both sides. Place them on a warm frying pan or griddle.

5. Fry them on each side for 1-4 minutes, depending on how you like your steak.

6. Once they've been fried, feel free to place them on a bed of spinach or other vegetables.

7. Enjoy your meal!

Breakfast Burritos

Don't think that these recipes can only be utilized for dinner. Every single one of your meals can be transformed into something that's tasty *and* good for you. The following recipe is entirely customizable, so feel free to add, take away, and mix your own favorite ingredients. Additionally, the ingredients below are for 5 burritos, perfect for meal prepping for your week to come!

Here's what you'll need:

- 5 wholemeal tortillas

- 250g black beans

- 10 medium eggs

- 1 large white onion (chopped)

- 100g chopped tomatoes

- 150g brown rice

- 50g pickled and sliced jalapenos

- 1 tsp salt, black pepper, paprika

- 125g low fat cheddar

- 10 chopped pork sausages (or your protein of choice)

Directions:

1. Boil the rice. This can be done by pouring the rice into a saucepan full of cold water. Bring to a boil, turn the heat to low, cover with a lid, and let simmer for 10 to 15 minutes. Add in the chopped tomatoes.

2. Drizzle a large non-stick pan with coconut oil. Add in the chopped onions and fry for 3-4 minutes. Take them off once they've been browned.

3. Add the cut up sausage and black beans. Fry these for 3-4 minutes until they are crispy. Once complete, put them in a bowl and set aside.

4. Next, fry the eggs. Just as usual, crack the eggs into a bowl and whisk. Pour the mixture into the pan and fry for 3-4 minutes.

5. Now, lay your burritos flat on a counter or table. Divide the rice in a short line running down the middle. Add the rest of the ingredients in any order you wish.

6. Wrap your burritos, tucking the bottom ends inside. Feel free to fry these gently as well or eat them right away.

<u>Chicken Pasta Salad</u>

This following recipe is a simple and delicious lunch recipe that is full of protein and essential nutrients. A meal like this will give you energy to exercise while also satisfying your hunger. You won't even notice this is a time-efficient, healthy meal! Here's what you'll need for 3 servings:

For the pasta:

- 160g cooked pasta

- 2 stalks celery

- 3 cooked chicken breasts

- 1 yellow pepper

- 2 tbsp low fat ranch dressing (or whatever dressing you choose)

- 1 handful cherry tomatoes

- 1 large handful mixed greens

For the sauce:

- 175ml peri-peri sauce

- 4 tbsp butter

- Half a tsp garlic powder

- 1 pinch salt

Directions:

1. In a saucepan, over medium heat, cook the peri-peri sauce and garlic powder. After 2

minutes, add the butter and salt and cook together for 5 minutes. Remove and cool.

2. Once you have chopped your celery and tomatoes and shred the chicken, place into a large mixing bowl with the cooked pasta.

3. Drizzle the cool dressing on top and thoroughly mix.

4. Enjoy! It's that easy!

Super Oats

Now, if you are someone who enjoys dessert now and then, or even a snack in between meals, this is the recipe for you. As previously mentioned, low fat and high protein foods aren't just for dinner. This porridge can be eaten for breakfast or for dessert; this is what you'll need:

- 75g dairy-free yogurt

- 1 tsp cinnamon

- 1 tbsp almond butter (or your nut butter of choice)

- 125ml almond milk (or your milk of choice)

- 50g instant oats

- Pinch salt

Directions:

1. Simply mix all these ingredients into a large cup or mug.

2. Cover and refrigerate for at least 4 hours, or overnight

3. Take out and enjoy! Eat with a spoon or straw!

As you can see, eating plenty of protein while maintaining an extensive workout routine is entirely possible. Each one of these meals will supply you with your necessary intake of fiber, amino acids, omega fatty acids, and various vitamins and minerals. These are the elements that will help you go out and exercise while still keeping you satisfied.

If you currently have a vastly different diet, slowly incorporate these meals into your daily menu. Before you know it, eating a lean and healthy diet will be a common occurrence for you.

Remember, losing weight doesn't need to be about dieting and limiting the intake of foods you love. You can still lose weight and gain muscle while enjoying the things you love. It's all a matter of increasing your intake of healthy foods and getting sufficient physical activity.

Additionally, if there is an ingredient you don't like, substitute it. Customize these recipes to your liking, and you'll be well on your way towards a healthy lifestyle!

COOKING ON A BUDGET

Many people get intimidated by whole food, clean eating due to the price tag often associated with it. However, you can lead a healthy life without breaking the bank. There are plenty of ways to cut costs while cooking at home, many of which you may not be aware of.

There are many habits, tips, and tricks that you can easily add to your daily routine to ensure you don't spend more than you need to.

Versatile Ingredients

First, try to buy ingredients that are versatile. A great example of this would be a simple rotisserie chicken. Rotisserie chickens take no time to prepare and are full of healthy fats and protein.

First, pick off all the meat off of the chicken. You can use these pieces in a number of ways: You can make shredded chicken sandwiches, chicken salad, casseroles, and more. If you really want to save time, meal prep for the next few days. Separate these chicken pieces the following breakfasts, lunches, and dinners.

Once you have picked off the chicken, do not throw away the bones. These bones can then be utilized to make chicken stock! Making chicken broth only takes a few minutes: toss the bones in a large pot with a couple of liters of water. Add in some chopped onions, garlic, and other seasonings. Let them simmer together for about an hour, and you're done! It's that simple.

Another example of a versatile ingredient is eggs. Eggs can be eaten for breakfast, lunch, dinner, or snacks, depending on how you prepare them. They go well with vegetables, fruit, in sandwiches or salads.

A container of a dozen eggs will cost you around $2. Learn how to make use of such a cost-efficient ingredient! One egg will have about 100 calories and 6 grams of protein, making them the perfect thing to eat when trying to lose some weight. Eggs and steamed vegetables make a great, cheap meal- that's tasty too!

It's important to figure out ways to use large or inexpensive ingredients in a multitude of ways. Oftentimes, we throw out valuable pieces of our food that could be later. Learn how to make use out of everything that you have. Doing so will ensure that we save money *and* time.

Consume Less Meat

The next tip is about learning to find protein in sources other than meat. As we now know, consuming protein is vital to gaining muscle mass. However, meat is expensive, and eating it every day is not recommended. Many people think protein is synonymous with animal meat, but that is simply not the case.

If you want to cut down on your meat consumption, there are other ways you can eat protein. Eggs, beans, yogurt, seeds, and nuts are great sources of protein. When making meatloaf or even tacos, try substituting some of the meat with beans. This will cost you less and provide you with sufficient fiber to your diet.

Walnuts, cashews, pistachios, sunflowers seeds, and chia seeds are just some of the nuts and seeds you can consume throughout your day without breaking the bank. Additionally, adding nut butters, such as almond or peanut butter, are a great way to consume quick protein.

The goal isn't to cut out meat from your diet entirely. Instead, just reduce your consumption with substitutions and alternatives. Meat can appear on your plate without taking up so much space. Meat can be used as a garnish or condiment, not necessarily as the star of the meal. Purchasing less meat will not only save you money, but will foster a healthy diet too.

Know Where to Go

Sometimes what you buy is just as important as where you buy it. Learning about the supermarkets, grocery stores, and specialty stores in your area will mean you always have a place to go for what you need.

For spices and dried peppers, try out your local ethnic grocery store. Asian markets with butchers or meat freezer sections will always have cheaper cuts of meat. Delis are a great place to get a plethora of sausages and wursts for a fraction of the price at a chain grocery store.

Don't think that the prices listed on a particular item are the cheapest they can be. If you find out that one store has better deals than another, divide your shopping list depending on location. Go to one grocery store for meat, and another for grains, for example.

Figure out which stores have their deals and which offer rewards and points. Take advantage of these systems to save your wallet on high-quality items. Some people even recommend doing your major shopping on Wednesdays, for this is when the sales from the previous weekend and the new ones begin. You can even solely shop in the evenings when perishables are discounted.

Lastly, buy what is in season. In today's world, it is possible to buy certain fruits and vegetables when they aren't in season- however, that isn't always cost-efficient. Instead, head to your local farmer's market and buy what is in season. Not only will they cost less, but they will also be fresher and better for you!

Meal Prep

Lastly, make meal prepping a habit. As previously mentioned, meal prepping is a great way to save money and time on your day to day meals.

Amidst living hectic, fast paced lives, it can be difficult to invest a lot of time into home cooking. Especially when aiming to eat healthily, it can be hard to avoid take out and fast food when we simply don't have the time. Meal prepping is a great tool to ensure that no matter where you are, or how busy, there will always be a delicious healthy meal waiting for you.

Meal prepping does require planning and organizing beforehand, but for such a small time commitment, it really pays off in the long run.

First, create a menu for your week (or month). Ideally, this would include breakfast, lunch, dinner, and snacks in between—next, figure out what ingredients you will need for every meal. Write out a detailed grocery list and hit the aisles. This method will ensure that you not only buy in bulk, but you buy everything you need at once (will limit your trips to the grocery store significantly!).

Next, devote one day to cooking the majority of your meals. It is a good idea to focus on foods that will take the longest to cook. Foods such as chicken, fish, rice, quinoa, and roasted vegetables are what you should start on first. You can also start preparing staple foods that are easy to add to meals or great to eat on their own. Hard-boiled eggs, chopped fruit, and washed greens are examples.

To save even *more* time, learn how to effectively

multi-task! While foods are baking or boiling, start chopping vegetables or washing greens for another meal. When you meal prep, you will quickly learn that there is always something that needs to be done.

If you find a recipe that you like, make extra portions for meals later in the week. Start freezing, canning, or storing these foods to ensure that they stay fresh for longer. Make sure to label every container so you know when things were made when they were opened and when they should be eaten by.

Once you have completed your meals, section them off into containers for later. It's ok if there are some dishes that will require some cooking later on; not everything can be made beforehand. Store these containers in the fridge or pantry.

Meal prepping may seem time intensive for a beginner, but soon you will notice how much free time you have during the week. Doing all your shopping, cooking, and preparing in one day means the rest of your days are free!

There is no right method to meal prepping; you will need to do it a few times to figure out what works best for you. If you are trying to lose weight, prepping each meal in advance ensures that there is no chance for you to over or under eat.

When setting up portion sizes, you can even organize your plate, so you are always eating a well-balanced meal- no matter the time of day. Ultimately, making meal prepping a habit will ensure that you save time and money, all while enjoying healthy, homemade foods.

There are plenty of tips, tricks, and habits you can learn to reduce your spending costs. Home Cooking doesn't need to be a stressful experience. It can be cheap, easy, and incredibly rewarding; all it takes is forethought and preparation.

HOW TO STAY IN SHAPE OVERSEAS

It can be relatively easy to stay on track when you're at home, but maintaining a healthy lifestyle while traveling can be a whole other challenge.

It is not uncommon for people to gain weight and lose track of their fitness when they are overseas. It is entirely normal to want to explore unique cuisines, foods, and drinks. After all, vacations are a time for us to sit back and relax. However, there are plenty of ways you can still enjoy yourself while remaining on top of your health.

Stay Active

When most people think of a workout routine, they picture a gym with weight machines and treadmills. Don't spend your vacation looking for a gym or workout space. Instead, learn the ways you can exercise *wherever* you are.

There are plenty of routines and activities that do not require special gear or equipment. Most of the time, all you will need is your body and some motivation.

Look back to Chapter 1: Simple Warmups. None of these warm ups require any objects or gear. Take advantage of this list and adopt them into your routine overseas. All you will need is some space to move freely.

Once you have warmed up, you can get creative. You can do pull ups on a tree branch or playground, push ups literally anywhere, and weightlifting with anything you have on hand (suitcases are great!). Being away from home should never be an excuse to slack off.

If you *can* bring one piece of exercise equipment, a resistance band is recommended. This little piece of equipment is small and easy to pack. It can easily be tucked into your bag and pulled out whenever you need it. Resistance bands offer a wide variety of workouts and can easily increase the intensity of your routine.

Additionally, staying active doesn't need to *feel* like staying active. When traveling to a point of interest, try walking instead of taking public transport. This will allow you the opportunity to see the surrounding areas while getting in extra cardio. Many cities today have bike rentals that are available year round.

This is another easy way to keep your body moving while still enjoying the view. If distances are too far, try walking or biking half way, or partially. Any amount helps!

Instead of choosing to spend your day lounging at the beach, opt for more active activities to throw yourself into. Try hiking to a viewpoint, for example. You can even try out surfing, kayaking, beach volleyball, or rock climbing. Get a sense of the country's culture by learning how the locals spend their time outdoors. Swimming or snorkeling are two other great ways to explore the local wildlife while also getting your body moving.

Even if for half an hour a day, doing such activities will get your endorphins flowing and your heart pumping. Before you know it, you will feel better, look better, and *be* better.

Eat Smart

Being overseas means being exposed to a beautiful array of exciting foods and flavors. While this should be a time to be adventurous, you should also make sure you are eating smart.

Your diet is 80% of the battle. Keep this in mind when you are tempted to eat a bowl of ice cream or order seconds. There are plenty of ways you can eat healthily and stay fit while traveling.

If you are staying at a hostel or at a place with a kitchenette, try cooking at least one meal a day. Breakfast is usually the easiest. When you are in complete control of the ingredients that go into your meals, the less chance there will be for you to cheat.

Spend some time buying groceries the day before and enjoy a homemade breakfast in the morning. Not only will this save you some extra cash, restaurants, and store-bought foods are usually higher in calories.

Try making some porridge for a quick and hearty breakfast. Even a simple salad with fruits is a great energy boosting option for a quick morning meal. Making this a habit will ensure that you are in control of what you are putting into your body at the start of every day.

Of course, it won't be possible to make your own food for every meal. But that doesn't mean you can't eat smart. When dining out, try ordering a dish but splitting it with someone to prevent overindulging.

Or, you can even order a small dish, and if you're still hungry after, order a second one. This ensures that you never over eat. And if you ever do get full, you can always ask for it to be wrapped up to be eaten later.

Don't be afraid to ask questions. Most restaurants are accommodating with certain ingredients and garnishes. You can always ask how something is made or what it is prepared with.

Deep fried items can be swapped out for fresh vegetables, and dressings can be served on the side. Asking questions ensures that you always know what is going into your body.

Why It's Important

There's no question why people add a few inches to their waistband when traveling; it's a time to let go. For some, enjoying a vacation means forgoing healthy lifestyle routines. It may seem like not exercising, and eating whatever you want for only two weeks won't make a difference. But stopping your routine completely can reap negative effects on your body.

These effects may not be easy to spot while you're away, but when you're back at home, you will notice. Your body takes time to adjust to whatever routine you put it through. When you take time off, getting back in shape will be harder to do, and more time consuming. It's always easier to continue staying in shape than to stop and start again over and over.

When you stop using your muscles, they depreciate. Athletes, for example, can start losing muscle mass just after three weeks of inactivity. You lose cardiovascular fitness even faster; this can take only a few days to reduce.

Additionally, don't shock your body with new foods. If you spent a lot of time reducing your intake of meat, for example, don't start eating meat at every meal. Your body can go into shock with new flavors, compounds, and nutrients. Instead, add new foods into your diet slowly and carefully. Always treat your body with respect because it will always react to mistreatments.

After putting in so much effort into your health and wellbeing, it doesn't make sense just to throw it all away. If you don't want to lose your muscle mass and fitness, keep active while overseas using the tips listed above.

That doesn't mean you need to maintain your usual exercise routine. Make sure you keep realistic goals. Instead, exercise just enough so that nothing starts depreciating. This can be as easy as taking part in the various aforementioned outdoor activities.

Keep your normal diet in mind, and try to stick to it. Traveling overseas can be a healthy and enriching experience as long as you are deliberate with your lifestyle choices.

Relax

Traveling should be an exciting and enriching time for you, so don't fret over the little things. Worrying over every little calorie and pound can ruin an entire vacation. It's entirely okay if you have one or two cheat meals, or you don't exercise as much as you planned. The most important thing is that you are enjoying yourself and the company of others.

It can be easy to get caught up in our health when we're away from home. You don't need to go overboard, just do what you need in order to feel healthy. Stress will always make it harder to lose weight and stay on track, remember that.

HOW TO STAY MOTIVATED

Everyone faces challenges when trying to reach a healthy lifestyle. Some people deal with time management; others struggle with bad habits. Most of the time, whatever issue you are facing can be resolved with thorough mental training.

People say mind over matter, and this phrase couldn't be more true when talking about keeping up a happy and healthy lifestyle. Training yourself to remain positive and motivated in any circumstance will propel you forward and help you reach your goals.

In order to reach this mental state, all you need is focus and determination...

Exercising isn't easy for everyone; in fact, everyone struggles when first starting out. Staying healthy with proper exercise and a healthy diet doesn't ever become entirely easy- but your outlook on those limitations does.

Change Your Perspective

The way you look at your new lifestyle will greatly alter how difficult it seems to you. Instead of thinking like a couch potato, start thinking like an athlete. This may seem like a large jump to you, but it's easier than you think.

Start looking at your exercise as a privilege, not a hindrance. Think of how lucky you are to be able to move your body freely and make it stronger. You have a duty to keep your body healthy and happy.

Look at your future and ask yourself what you see. Do you see yourself overweight, unhappy, and sitting on the couch? Or do you see yourself fit, happy, and enjoying the outdoors with your family? Only you can decide which future you will have.

It's important not only to rely on yourself for motivation but to look to others for inspiration. Everyone you meet has something to offer, even those who are unable to be physically active. This will remind you how lucky you are to be able to go out and run and keep your body in shape. A fitness routine doesn't start at the gym; it starts in your head. Don't focus on all the things you will be losing; look at all the things you will be gaining instead.

Set Goals

No one runs without a finish line in the distance. It will always be harder for you to exercise if there isn't a place you're trying to reach. Instead of working out aimlessly, set yourself a goal.

Fitness goals can look different to different people. You can have a goal of losing ten pounds, you can have a goal of running 5 kilometers, or you can have a goal of doing 100 push ups. You can even have a goal of fitting into your old jeans again. Whatever your goal is, visualizing it in your mind will give you purpose and keep you motivated.

Remember to set realistic goals. Don't aim to run a marathon next week when you just started jogging today. Your life should be able to accommodate these new goals, not shut down for them. If you don't set practical goals, you'll be setting yourself up for failure.

This is when you will want to give up. It's common for people to quit when they feel like they aren't making any progress. Make sure you note even the smallest achievements so you can clearly see how much you have improved. Don't expect to reach your goal overnight; everything takes time and effort. Understand that this commitment is long term; the benefits will only come with sustained hard work.

Try writing down your goal in a highly visible place. Revisit it often, so you don't forget. Let this mantra reinforce your effort and remind you why you are doing this in the first place. You can even try to visualize your goal before every workout. Picture this future in your mind, and it will push you to keep going.

Keep It Fresh

No one likes getting stuck in a boring routine. This can make our lives feel stagnant and repetitive. By nature, we need variety in order to stay motivated during long term efforts.

Make sure you switch up your exercises now and then to keep things fresh. Sometimes, even a change in scenery can make all the difference. You can alternate between working out in the gym and working out in a park. You can even set aside one day in your routine when you will swim, or bike, or go on a hike instead of using equipment.

Our day to day lives change more than we think.

Your exercise routine should reflect that. Alter your routine for the changing seasons, and for your work week.

In addition to keeping your fitness fresh, you should also keep it fun. No one said working out had to be something that you dread every week- it can also be something you genuinely look forward to.

Try to include activities that make you forget that you're exercising. Dancing with friends and group sports are great ways to move your body in a fun way. Soon enough, your workout won't seem like a chore; it will seem like just another hobby.

Changing up your routine now and then doesn't only keep you motivated, it helps your body. Trying out different movements and activities introduces you to new muscle groups you may have been neglecting. Some exercises work out your back, while others work out your legs- it's important to do both.

Look to Others

As previously mentioned, encouragement can be found anywhere. If you feel like you're always exercising while others are sitting at home, or you're always eating salad while others are eating cake, look for a friend. Try to find someone whose values and goals align with yours. Working hard will always seem easier when you feel like you're in it with someone else.

You can run with this person once a week. They will push you to keep going when you're tired, and you'll do the same for them. Having a partner will also keep you accountable. If you set a certain schedule for your workouts together, you will be less inclined to cancel. When someone depends on your participation, you'll think twice before hitting the snooze button.

If you can't find someone like this, try looking online. Today there are countless communities, forums, and sites full of trainers, experts, and like minded individuals. Go to them every time you need support. When we feel lifted up by a community, we are more likely to strive towards our goals.

Changing your perspective, setting realistic goals, keeping it fresh, and looking to others will keep you on track. We all feel discouraged at some point. Even the people who you look up to struggled to get where they are now. Remember that results will only come to those who work for them.

Understand that though others may support you, positivity and motivation can only come from within. No one can do the work for you; you need to be the one to take the initiative. Only you can decide what goals to set and what schedule to keep to. You need to work little by little to learn what works best for you and your lifestyle. Take responsibility for your health, and you'll never turn back. The ideal future that's waiting for you is there for the taking; all you need to do is reach out and grab it.

Never give up

What if I get in trouble? What if something doesn't work out the way it should?

It's happened to me too. But it's normal, there is no one method that is 100% effective for everyone.

But as we have seen, mine is not a method, I mean, I don't have a magic formula, but I am simply giving you the knowledge and tools to achieve your goal.

Most people will get great results right away and in a short time, they will reach the goal they have set themselves.

A small percentage will encounter greater difficulties, perhaps few or no results in the first few weeks, but that's where you won't have to give up, because there are those who, for various reasons, have a particularly stuck metabolism.

One of the main reasons why people fail and give up everything is the self-conception that nothing will ever work.

It's not easy, but this is what you have to do...:

- Think positive: you' ve certainly achieved some benefit, focus on that.

- Roll up your sleeves and keep training by increasing the intensity of the exercise. If, on the contrary, you continue at the same pace, the results will unfortunately be the same...

- Do not lose hope and confidence in yourself (and in me)

OPERATING MATERIAL: EXAMPLE OF TABLES.

Monitoring Table

Number of Weeks	Waist in cm	Waist Variation	Around the chest in cm	Chest-to-Breast Variation	Around the thigh in Cm	Around the thigh variation	% of Fat Mass	Fat Mass Variation
0								
1								
2								
3								
4								
5								
6								

Calculate your fat mass in % using, I remind you, the formulas I indicated earlier.

First, you will have to measure the required circumferences.

Instructions on how best to take measurements:

Get a measuring tape and stand in front of a mirror and:

1. Measure your waist: with a measuring tape, measure the narrowest point of the waist, usually a few inches above the navel.

2. Measure your waistline: in this case, measure the widest point, usually just above the nipples.

3. For the thigh, it is ideal to take the measurement on the groin following the line of the pelvis passing through the buttocks..

PLAN YOUR FEEDING WEEK

	MON	TUES	WED	THUR	FRI	SAT	SUN
BREAKFAST							
SNACK							
MORNING							
LUNCH							
SNACK							
AFTERNOON							

TRAINING: SCHEDULE YOUR WEEK

	MON	TUES	WED	THUR	FRI	SAT	SUN
WORKOUT ROUTINES							
AEROBIC TRAINING							
TIMETABLE							

MANAGEMENT TRAINING

Create a similar table with your favorite editor or create the table by hand.

Put an X or type Yes in the box of the corresponding day and training. Don't underestimate the "time" row: it is essential that you give yourself precise RULES, so "set" the time of each workout.

I found it essential to avoid procrastinating the time of training during the day, perhaps by improvising it, at a time of the day when you have little time.

You risk training badly and incompletely.

You can do all this in digital format or print and write it manually.

CONCLUSIONS

When you've finally overcome all the difficulties and seen the incredible results of my training with your own eyes, you'll be able to show off a beautifully sculpted physique and your abs without being ashamed of your unattractive belly.

You'll improve your posture and have many other positive sensations: you'll feel as light as a feather and capable of any physical activity.

You will certainly feel more confident, increase your self-esteem and be more successful in relationships.

Ok, in this book, I have given you THE best solution I have ever used to sculpt my abs and of those who trusted me.

But now it's your turn!

It's your turn. Get in the game and start practicing what you've learned in this report right now:

- Take a measuring tape and measure the circumferences to find out what % of your body fat mass is. Write it down in a table and calculate it.

- Set the workout that suits you best and program it weekly, do the same thing with regard to nutrition using the tables in the **Operating Material.**

- Learn how to feed yourself properly.

- Do it now.

If you do everything right, you'll see that the results won't be long in coming and in a very short time, you'll have achieved your final result.

I wish you to achieve exactly the result you are visualizing in your head.

If you liked this Book, leave me a 5 Stars on Amazon

Your opinion is very important to me. In recognition of the value of the information I gave you, you can leave me a nice 5-star review.

If on the contrary, you have any doubts, do not hesitate to contact me and encourage me to improve. I want to satisfy those who trust me.

Write to my personal email massimo@fitnessmax.it with subject "Perplexity book Workout Routines for Men".

Thank you!

See you soon,

Massimo

Other Useful Resources

I will soon update this section with the other books. This is the first.

My Italian website www.fitnessmax.it